WHAT YOUR CHILD NEEDS TO KNOW
ABOUT SEX (AND WHEN)

WHAT YOUR CHILD NEEDS TO KNOW ABOUT SEX (AND WHEN)

A STRAIGHT-TALKING GUIDE FOR PARENTS

DR. FRED KAESER

Foreword by JEANNE ELIUM

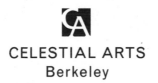

CELESTIAL ARTS
Berkeley

Library of Congress Cataloging-in-Publication Data

Kaeser, Fred.
  What your child needs to know about sex and when : a straight-talking guide for
parents / Fred Kaeser.
     p. cm.
  Summary: "A straight-talking guide for modern parents about how and
when to talk to their young children about sex and sexuality, from a
professor of human sexuality and former director of health for New York
City public schools"—Provided by publisher.
  Includes bibliographical references and index.
  1. Sex instruction for children. 2. Children and sex. I. Title.

HQ57.K34 2011
649'.65—dc22

2011009689

ISBN 978-1-58761-250-3

Printed in the United States of America

Cover design by Betsy Stromberg
Interior design by Colleen Cain

10 9 8 7 6 5 4 3 2 1

First Edition

CONTENTS

FOREWORD

Early in my parenting career, I remember looking at my children in alarm after a particularly vexing incident and thinking, "I don't know what to do next!" Many times I wished that sons and daughters came with individual instruction books, listing in simple directions the most propitious thing to do and say in any challenging situation. That wish never went away as my kids progressed through each childhood phase with me working to keep one step ahead of them. In lieu of a stork-delivered set of guidelines, I turned to the experts' "how-to's" for guidance. All good advice, these self-help books outlined how important it was to talk so my kids would listen, to set limits and boundaries, to avoid unnecessary battles, and to follow through on what I said would happen if they failed to follow through. Heady stuff, and that's where a lot of the information stayed—in my head—until I learned to take a deep breath, slow down, and consider before I took action. Simply saying "Let me think about that" gave me more time and less cause to regret my answers and actions.

But, then there was the issue of sex. Though I consider myself as open about sex as the next educator, the thought of initiating "the talk" had me worried. I certainly had no helpful role model, as my mother simply handed me a book that discussed the mating habits of animals with a look that said, "Don't ask me." To say that the book disgusted me, even though I was a farm kid, is putting it mildly. So when it came my turn to enlighten the next generation about sex, I was at a loss. When is the best time to introduce the topic? How detailed should I be? What words should I use?

I think I didn't do too badly, but how much easier our conversations might have gone had I had Dr. Kaeser's amazing guide for parents about what our children need to know about sex. Of course, times were different when my children were small—no cell phones, no Facebook, and for the most part no explicit sexual scenes on TV. I didn't have to work as hard as today's parents to counter the exposure to an oversexualized culture. Indeed, I am rather astonished at Dr. Kaeser's assertion that sexuality issues are affecting younger and younger children. Had you asked me at what age a parent should talk to a child about sex, I would have answered that it depends on the child. "Not so," says Dr. Kaeser, with a doctoral degree in human sexuality studies from New York University and whose many years of experience in talking with parents and children about sexual matters makes him an expert extraordinaire. He emphasizes that to keep our children safe, it's never too early but that it can be too late to talk about sex. In a culture where ten is the new sixteen in regards to sexuality, he admonishes that adolescence is far too late to introduce the topic of sex.

In an open and personable style, Dr. Kaeser suggests what information to give and when to give it based on age and gender. He uses all of "the words" with humor, reassurance, hard facts, and helpful examples. Most importantly, he advocates that parents use teachable moments to convey not only the specifics but also moral values. The "Big Three"—love, respect, and trust—figure repeatedly in this well-written book, persuading parents to define and clarify their own values and feelings about sexual issues. Dr. Kaeser puts the responsibility for educating our children about sex where it should be, squarely on the shoulders of parents. We don't have to do it alone, however, because his approachable book is designed to make us informed, approachable parents. I wish he had written *What Your Child Needs to Know About Sex (and When)* thirty years earlier!

Jeanne Elium
Walnut Creek, California
May 2011

ACKNOWLEDGMENTS

I would like to thank Sharon Bowers of the Miller Agency for telling me I should write this book and Cindy Nye, my wife, for making me. And Lara Naaman for getting me started. Of course, this book would never have been done without Ten Speed Press. Julie Bennett saw the need for a book like this and Sara Golski helped me make it happen. Thanks as well to Ron Moglia and Derek Calderwood of NYU for teaching me well. I wouldn't have the sex education experience I do if it wasn't for the New York City Department of Education allowing me to work with all the students and parents through the years. Tony Alvarado and Marjorie Robbins, you both allowed me to take risks and push the envelope. And of course, my son Bret, who showed me exactly how an adolescent can be responsible and trustworthy.

INTRODUCTION

Congratulations! By opening this book, you've moved one step closer to becoming an approachable parent for your child on all matters sexual.

I'm Fred Kaeser, former director of health for the New York City Department of Education, and I'd like to speak to you about your child's sexuality. It's pretty frightening out there these days, isn't it? If you're the parent of a child who is twelve, eleven, or ten years of age—or even younger—this is your book. You know all too painfully well just how crazy this hypersexualized world is, and how it is affecting your child and other young children. (If your child is already in middle school, know that although I focus here on somewhat younger children, you should keep reading; there's plenty in here that will be of help to you.)

Perhaps your six-year-old has come home from school asking what *sexy* means, because he has heard other kids using the term. Or perhaps your seven-year-old son's friend forcefully touched your boy's penis on a play date, and your boy has come to you frightened and upset. Or maybe your ten-year-old wants to create a profile on Facebook or MySpace, and you want to say no, but you're afraid that if you do it'll cause a nasty confrontation.

You are certainly not alone in your concerns. Today, sexuality-related issues are affecting younger and younger children. No matter your culture, religion, ethnicity, race, or socioeconomic status, if you live in

1

America you are dealing with a sexually saturated society that bombards young children with sexual messages. These messages—many of which are explicit, heterosexist, homophobic, and misogynistic—have invaded our homes, our schools, our playgrounds, and our communities like never before. The innocent days of *Leave It to Beaver* are long gone, and all parents, regardless of their child's age, are confronted with the harsh reality that they *must* become sex educators for their children. We cannot put off conversations about sex and sexuality or hope that our schools and places of worship will take on this responsibility. We must stand up and face this reality head-on.

Parents of young children are being forced to confront sexual behaviors and concerns that no previous generation of parents has had to deal with. This means that we must be prepared to discuss certain aspects of sex and sexuality with our children at ages that seem far too young for this. It means that before middle school—indeed, by age ten—we must be having conversations about intercourse: what it really is, and when is the right time to have it, with whom, and under what conditions. We must discuss with our children why people have sex and why some people try to hurt other people through sex. We must explain to them why they are too young to join Facebook, MySpace, and other social networking sites. We must talk with them about kids who molest other kids. We have to talk about contraception and condoms, and how to protect themselves from sexually transmitted diseases. In short, everything that you thought your sixteen-year-old had to know about sex is what your ten-year-old now needs to know. We have been witnessing this "age creep," with regard to the age at which a young person must become informed about human sexuality, for several generations now. As the world around us becomes increasingly more sexually explicit, there is the accompanying need for parents to address the complexities of sexuality with their children at younger and younger ages. Consequently, ten is the new sixteen!

But there is some good that emerges from this craziness. If we take the responsibility to have these meaningful discussions with our children about sex and sexuality by the time they are ten years of age, there is a good chance we will see some remarkable, positive results. If we do this, it is likely that our kids will make the following choices:

- Postpone intercourse until adulthood (When I say adulthood, I mean some point over the age of eighteen. I will describe in detail later on the various qualities I believe one must possess prior to engaging in sexual intercourse—and age is only one of them. While there is no guarantee that the older a person is when they have sex, the less risk they will experience, it is reasonable to suggest that someone nineteen, twenty, or older will make better sexual decisions than a teen would.)

- Avoid getting pregnant or contracting a sexually transmitted disease during adolescence

- Avoid sexually abusive relationships

- Above all, develop a healthy attitude toward sexuality

It really is that simple. If you win the battle to become the number one influence on your child's sexual behavior, you will see these remarkable results. Forget school sex education; forget community-based support programs; forget trying to fight the media's sexualization of everything. If we do our job correctly, we win. If we don't—and right now many of us are not managing this crucial task—then we lose out to our child's peers, the media, and all the other influences clamoring to capture our kids' heads and hearts.

If you communicate with your child early and often about sex, are authentic and sincere in your discussions, and do so as part of an authoritative style of parenting, you and your child are going to be just fine. You'll find that you can do a better job of influencing your child's sexual behavior than any educational program. That's how powerful an influence we parents can be on our children. This is not rocket science; you don't need a PhD to make this happen. I'll say it again: *Parents can be the most significant influence on children's sexual behavior.*

Yet even though we can wield more influence over our children than any other entity they encounter, somewhere along the way many of us have become lost in our efforts to effectively parent in this hypersexualized world. After all, for the most part, us parents have grown up "sex stupid." By this I mean not that we are actually stupid, but that we have had a woefully inadequate preparation to be "sex smart." Now we live in a world that is sex saturated. No wonder many parents either don't feel confident communicating with their children about sex or would rather have someone else teach their children.

So we're going to sit down on the couch together, you and I, and figure this whole thing out. It'll be just you and me, parent to parent. You're going to learn what to say, how to say it, and when to say it. I'm going to make this as easy to understand as possible. I'm not going to recommend any books your child can read about sex; I'm not going to suggest any educational videos or DVDs that you could show your child; there will be no props, no gimmicks, and no gadgets. This is all about you, the parent, becoming approachable for your child.

I hear doubts from parents all the time: *It's so hard; my kid won't listen to me; I can't get through to her; I can't compete with his friends, the media, or the Internet; there's sex all around us.* It goes on and on. I'm here to tell you, you *can* do it. Have faith in yourself. And I'll be there with you along the way.

I hear another concern: *All this talking about sex will make my kids more curious or even make them go and try it out.* But you'll find that just the opposite happens—particularly when you learn how to package your conversations around sex. You're going to be sharing your values and helping your child understand what is right and wrong with regard to certain sexual behavior, and you're going to be authentic and sincere in your discussions. That is, you're going to help your children understand how to manage real-life situations they may encounter as they learn about relationships and sexual behavior. And you'll use a style of parenting that sets clear and defined boundaries for behavior: you'll be an authoritative parent.

Why listen to me? What makes me an authority on such matters? Well, I may have fielded more questions about sex and had more conversations about sex with kids of all different ages than any other adult, ever! In fact, I have been a sexual educator and director of health for more than twenty-five years in the largest public school system in the United States. I have held various positions, including director of health education for 1,300 schools and director of health services for 260 schools. Over the years, I have been asked by teachers and principals to speak to children and adolescents about sexuality. I have spoken to thousands of elementary, middle, and high school students, but I confess I've always preferred speaking to elementary students. My favorite age group has always been ten- and eleven-year-olds—that is, fifth-grade students. At these ages, most children are either on the cusp of or just beginning puberty, basically very innocent and wide eyed, but also very hungry for information and guidance about sex. I have found that when you have truthful, dignified, and adult-like conversations with them about sexuality, they just eat it up! Kids appreciate it when an adult shows them the respect they deserve by helping them better understand the sexualized world that is all around them.

I have a doctoral degree in human sexuality studies from New York University, and over the years I've studied the modern problem of the accelerating premature sexualization of young people. I have given hundreds of presentations to school PTAs and parent groups on the topic of communicating with children about sexuality, and have consulted with many individual parents who had sexual concerns about their children. Many school principals, administrators, and counselors have asked me to intervene and assist with problematic sexual behaviors of children and adolescents, many of which were actually taking place in their schools. My work along these lines has provoked my concern, in particular, over a problem that has emerged since the 1990s: the apparent increase in sexual bullying and molestation of children by other children.

I am also a parent and have been married for thirty-five years. Two of the greatest challenges for any person—being an effective parent and maintaining a nurturing and caring lifelong partnership—have certainly given me invaluable insights for my professional role as a sexual educator. For all of us, our past experiences of learning about sex and sexuality help shape who we are as sexual beings today; so, too, have my personal experiences as a parent and a partner contributed greatly to my professional role as a sexual educator. I have often referred to these personal experiences during my work with students, parents, and school faculty. You will see these references throughout this book.

I have no doubt that as you read through this book you will have very strong opinions about what I say. Hopefully, you will agree with me, but there may be times when you don't. I do know, however, that my words and advice will challenge you to become the very best sex educator you can be for your children. You will find that as you read each chapter you will not only be evaluating what I am saying, but most importantly you will be thinking about what it is you need to do and say to help your child navigate this very sexualized world. So let us begin our journey together as you explore how to become an approachable parent for your child on all sexual matters.

CHAPTER 1

The Wall of Sexualized Messages

Sexual images and messages are everywhere these days. In your average day, how long is it before you are exposed to some sort of sexualized message? Television, music, billboards, print media, Internet, telephone and communication devices, cable, movies—there are just so many mediums through which sex and sexuality can be depicted.

I'm fifty-eight, and I still cannot get over how many explicit depictions of sexuality there are all around us today. I remember when I was fourteen, thinking I had died and gone to heaven when I found a *Playboy* magazine. But for some young people now, a *Playboy* magazine is a fairly mild form of stimulation, like *National Geographic*, with its depictions of naked people from tribal cultures, was for me when I was a boy: it'll get your attention, but not for very long. Now kids can see actual sexual intercourse as often as they want just by turning on the computer. In homes where kids have unsupervised, unfiltered Internet access, a world of outrageous sex is only a few clicks away. In fact, they can see sexual intercourse in all its possible permutations, everything from your run-of-the-mill sexual intercourse to the weirdest, sickest, most deviant sex acts. Even in homes that have computer Internet filters, many kids can find ways around them or turn to other devices to access the Internet. And if it's not the Internet, then perhaps it's cable television or pay per view. There's plenty of sex to be had there. Although perhaps not as outrageous as the Internet, cable does provide a wide array of explicit sexual messages. Then there's your child's mobile phone that can be used for sending and receiving naked pictures of him and his friends, and social networking sites that may be offering any number of provocative images and messages.

Even if your child is only four or five years of age, you need to ask yourself just how much she is being influenced by the television that she's watching. She may not understand the sexual content she sees, but, believe me, she is absorbing it. And once she starts school there is no doubt that she will be influenced by other children she encounters there.

As you can see, there are plenty of opportunities to pick up sexual content via any number of electronic and communicative devices. Besides these devices, there are many additional sources of sexualized messages that young kids can be exposed to today. Music offers an interesting array of sexualized possibilities as pop stars sing about sexual relationships and hookups, intermingled with hurtful and demeaning lyrics about women. Combined with video, they offer an extremely compelling genre that can overwhelm the senses with stimulating messages about sex, sexuality, and gender. Print media, including magazines, books, newspapers, and advertisements of all kinds, certainly offer any number of possibilities for exposure to sexual matters. And of course interactions with peers offer even more.

Our children have countless opportunities for exposure to sexual messages every day of their lives. Think about that—constant exposure to sexualized messages, day in and day out, at lightning speed from nearly every direction, for their entire childhood. This exposure often occurs without the guidance and intervention from parents and caregivers that is necessary to help children sort through and make sense of it all. These messages are not only explicit but are also frequently violent in nature, awash in male dominant and female submissive imagery—misogynistic, heterosexist, and sensational. Make no mistake about it; your child *will* be exposed to an enormous amount of sex-related content no matter how hard you try to shield them from it.

Our society is creating a hypersexualized generation of kids. Children today are more likely to confront sexual stimuli on an earlier and more frequent basis than any prior generation of children. Consequently, they are more at risk for thinking and acting in a sexual manner before they are emotionally and developmentally ready.

Block by Block, Building the Wall of Sex

To help you appreciate what our children are up against, I've come up with a simple illustration. Visualize your child sitting at a table. On the floor around her are thousands of one-inch square blocks. Each block represents some sort of sexualized message. Perhaps it's something sexual that she hears from a friend, some sexual image or content from TV, or sexual lyrics in a song. It could be any type of message that has some sexual reference, whether it is fairly innocent and benign or explicit and incomprehensible. But every block represents some sexual message your daughter or son could encounter on any given day.

The first time your child is exposed to one of these sexualized messages, a block is placed on the table in front of her. With her second exposure to a sexualized message, another block is placed on the table next to the first block. With the third exposure a block is placed next to the second, and so on, until the row is, let's say, eighteen inches long. With the next exposure, a block is placed on top of the first block in the first row. This continues with each exposure to a sexualized message.

With eighteen more blocks in place, a third row begins. A wall of blocks starts to form.

Got the picture? Now imagine how high the wall would be after just one day. How many sexualized messages—blocks—would be on the table in front of your child? Obviously, the older your child, the higher the wall is likely to be, simply because we would expect an older child to have more varied experiences and hence more exposures to sexual messages. So how high would you expect the wall to be after a week? How about a month? Six months? A year? Ten years? If I were a betting man, I'd say that the top of the wall of sexualized messages facing your child extends way up into the sky, well out of our sight. So think about this: by the time your child begins to enter puberty, he or she has probably been exposed to thousands, if not tens of thousands, of sexualized messages. And how many of these sexualized messages will be problematic and conflict with your values system? How many of them will portray women as sexual objects and men as hunters, lusting for sex? How many of them will be heterosexist and homophobic? How many of them will portray sexual intimacy and behavior without any sense of responsibility or consequences? How many of them will portray sex as something we can all engage in without having to be in love? How many of them are incomprehensible and just outright confusing to your young child? How many of them come from sources that you would have a problem with?

A Closer Look at the Wall

All this sends a little shiver down your spine, right? And what will that wall of sexualized messages look like after your child has entered puberty and his or her sexual feelings and desires start being actualized, and peers begin to have more influence on your child than ever before? How high will it be then? And there your child sits, with a gigantic wall of sexualized messages staring her or him in the face. Our job as parents is to help our children make sense of that wall.

Now, how many of the blocks in that wall are yours or your partner's? Have your messages about sex even come close to countering all those that were harmful to your child? If you don't take it upon yourself to become the most influential source of sexual guidance for your children, their friends and peers or the media are very willing and capable of doing it for you. Do you want most of the blocks in your child's wall of sexualized messages to come from the media and your child's peers, or from you?

We know just how powerful the media and our children's peers can be in informing and influencing them about sex and sexuality. Study after study consistently tells us that peers and the media are at the top of the list of influential sources of sexual information.[1]

Sexual Messages from You

But let's start first with you, the parent. Exactly what sort of sexual messages do you send to your child? How many of your blocks in the wall are messages that have had a positive influence on your child? How many have been a negative influence and have only added to your child's confusion and misunderstanding? Do you tell your little boy to be strong, suck it up when it hurts, and be tough? Do you buy your daughter low-cut tops and short skirts, and let her wear makeup at the age of nine? Are you the parent who wants to be friends with your child, tends to avoid confrontation, and has difficulty setting boundaries and saying no?

Your Silence Speaks Volumes

During a recent presentation for parents at a school, a parent of a nine-year-old told me that her boy's best friend had an iPad and would frequently go to very explicit websites and show her son the images he found there.

She said she had overheard her son talking about it and had gone to him to discuss it. He had replied that he thought it was disgusting but no big deal. She asked me, in front of about a hundred other parents, "So, what should I do? Should I let him do this or should I say something?"

"Are you kidding me?" I said. "There is no way you should be letting this happen. Go to the other boy's parents and state your concern. If they don't agree with you, you shouldn't allow your son to see that boy anymore. You then need to help your child make sense of the explicit sexual material he was looking at."

Her response was, "But I don't want to end his friendship. He would be so upset."

On the one hand, I can understand her response. No parent wants to disappoint her child by possibly ending a friendship. Obviously, she needs to reason with the parents of her son's friend and try to get them to understand the seriousness of the situation: nine-year-olds should not be viewing sexually explicit material. My guess is they would agree and intervene with their child appropriately. But, should they resist her wishes, she may have to endure the possible pain of having to tell her child that he can no longer see his friend. As difficult as this may be, it pales in comparison to the risks involved in allowing one's nine-year-old son to view sexually explicit material.

We continued to have some more back and forth, this parent and I. Other parents chimed in and the prevailing consensus was that this parent needed to confront her son's friend's parents—remaining silent would not work. She agreed, and hopefully she was able to work things out. Based on what this parent told me during the presentation, let's take a look at the various messages that were added to her son's sexualized wall. We know for sure that her nine-year-old son has been exposed, probably a number of times, to highly explicit sexual behavior. We know that he knows his mother is aware of it and to date has not taken a stand. So a number of harmful blocks have been added to his wall. The boy now has to deal with the highly sexualized images on his own and has to make sense of why his mom hasn't really taken any action.

Being exposed to highly sexualized images can have an immense impact on a young child without the intervening help of an empathetic adult. I will have much more to say on this topic later in the book. For now, we can only hope that his mom will offset the negative effects of these blocks by intervening. I would hope that she would tell her son that he doesn't need to see people having sex, that sexual videos usually do not offer an accurate portrayal of adult sexuality, that she will talk to his friend's mom and ask her to stop his friend from viewing and showing off the sexually explicit sites, that she is always available to talk about what he's seen on the iPad, and that she's taking this action because she loves him.

The Effects of the Wall: A Hypersexualized Generation of Children

When I say that we are creating a hypersexualized generation of children, I mean that a significant number of children are actually demonstrating sexual interest and/or behavior at earlier ages than ever before in our society. Growing up in the United States today, kids are being exposed to sexual matters that were previously only in the purview of adults. The greater the exposure to children, the greater the consequences can be. When parents fail to counter and buffer the plethora of sexual stimuli that build a child's wall of sexualized messages, children are then left to their own devices to manage what they experience. When children are exposed to explicit sexual behavior, some of which may be incomprehensible to them, we can expect several things to occur. At the very least many will be confused; they will have difficulty making sense of and putting into proper perspective what they are exposed to. Some will actually try to act out or mimic what they have seen. Others, who may be already developing an intrusive or bullying persona, will begin to incorporate sexual behavior into their bullying behavior.

The biggest impact of hypersexualization is its overall looming effect on the day-to-day existence of kids. Sexuality becomes much more of a player than it should, irrespective of the child's age:

- The five-year-old learns to use the word *sex* without having any clue what it means.
- Some of his peers his age become overly curious and actually touch each other's genitals as opposed to just looking (as in "I'll show you mine if you show me yours"). (Children have a very normal curiosity about basic sex differences and similarities between genders. They don't typically extend that curiosity to actual touching of the genitals.)
- The eight-year-old asks questions about dildos and wants to know how a man can become a woman.
- The ten-year-old asks about rimming (licking a sex partner's anus) and is already close to being sexually active.

Our children's lives are becoming saturated with sexual images and innuendos. Seven-year-old girls are dressed by their parents in skimpy skirts, spaghetti-strap tops, and makeup. Little boys learn dance steps with thrusting and grinding movements intended for the bedroom. School attire guidelines allow plunging necklines and bare midriffs for girls, and for the boys there's nothing like showing their underwear with low-hanging pants.

I have been inundated the past ten years with so many cases of sexualized behavior among elementary school children that at times it felt as though my head was spinning—kids five, six, seven, or eight years of age touching genitals, forcing other kids to do things that are sexual, or lying on top of each other, humping. Young kids have made sexual comments such as "I'm gonna sex you," "Let's play the sex game," and "Kiss my privates." You can ask any elementary school teacher who has been working with kids for any length of time, and I guarantee that he or she will tell you that there is more sexually related behavior and talk among students than ever before. Reading this right now, you may be thinking the same thing. You're saying to yourself that you've seen this kind of thing as well, or that you have a child who has experienced something similar.

Just fifteen or twenty years ago we saw this sort of behavior far more infrequently than we're seeing it now. We would have the occasional young student who would act out sexually, or we would see this behavior in kids who had been sexually abused. Now we are also seeing it in children who have been exposed to sexually explicit or incomprehensible sexual stimuli.

Let's think about the child whose wall of sexualized messages is constructed from numerous exposures to sexually explicit stimuli that he or she cannot comprehend. If this child's parents or guardians don't take enough time to talk with the child about sex and sexuality, and they do not adequately intervene when they know their child has been exposed (like the mother of the nine-year-old and the iPad), then it becomes increasingly likely that the child will begin to display some sort of problematic sexual behavior. This child might develop a preoccupation with sexual matters or themes, engage in repeated sexually explicit discussions with peers, or start to expose his or her genitals to others or attempt to view the genitals of others. Or perhaps this child will attempt to touch other children's genitals, or become sexually intrusive toward other children. These are just some of the concerns we have about a child who is confronted with excessively explicit and incomprehensible sexual messages. I will elaborate on these sorts of sexualized problems much more extensively in chapter 3.

Schools Offer Little Help

No other generation of children has been confronted with an overload of sexual stimuli of the scope and scale that we see today. As I said earlier, our society is both sex saturated and sex stupid. We apparently can't get enough sex in our daily lives, yet at the same time we spend countless hours debating whether or not children and adolescents should be taught sex education in our schools or by any source other than their parents. Think about this contradiction for a moment. Children are being exposed, day in and day out, to some incredibly wacky and bizarre sexual images and content, and are then passing this information on to other children, yet many parents are worried that school sex education will somehow contaminate their innocent minds with dangerous sexual information. Huh? What am I missing here? These parents argue that they want to be the ones to teach their child about sex and sexuality, and that they will be the ones to decide when it should be done. This would be fine, except a majority of parents profess to have considerable difficulty communicating with their children about sex and sexuality.[2] About one-third of us fear that talking to our kids about sex will cause them to have sex, another third feel uncomfortable, and the remaining third would prefer that others do the teaching for us. So many of us are really *not* doing what we claim we want to do—and we are leaving our children at the mercy of sexual misinformation.

Most parents actually want schools to teach sex education, but there's confusion over exactly what to teach and what values should be espoused. Nevertheless, most school districts in the country say they teach some form of sex education, although I would suggest it is usually at the high school level, with far less involvement at the middle and elementary school levels. Even when a school district says all of its schools teach sex education, it may not be comprehensive enough to have any meaningful, positive effect on young people's behavior. At the elementary school level, I would argue that the sex education programs are even less comprehensive. This represents perhaps the greatest tragedy because it is during elementary school that we can usually have the greatest effect on establishing positive behaviors. Even though study after study shows that a majority of parents in America support public school sex education, very few school districts can *honestly* say that their elementary school sex education is at the level necessary to positively affect the sexual behavior of its students.[3] I emphasize the word *honestly* because I know from firsthand experience how easy it is for a school district to inflate its positive numbers pertaining to sex or health education when surveyed by state government. A school district can report that it teaches sex education or health education when in reality it either doesn't come close to the scope and sequence that would make it worthy, or it offers it only in its secondary schools and not at the elementary level.

Of course, the great irony is that all schools have unofficial sex education programs, ones that are run by the students themselves during lunch period, during recess, in the school's bathrooms, and in the hallways during the changing of classes. Spend some time at a school and see for yourself the exchange of sexuality among its students. Students chatter about sex, text about sex, and sometimes actually engage in sex at school. Don't be shocked by what I say here. Schools offer an array of opportunities for students to express their sexuality. Far too many kids express sexual behaviors while at school. We know that a considerable amount of these behaviors are of an unwanted or hurtful nature, as is the case with forms of sexual harassment and misconduct.[4] But I also know firsthand that there are kids who will willingly engage in sexual behavior with each other in the more remote or private areas within a school building. Either way, it should be disturbing to all that any sort of sexual behavior occurs in schools.

So we have a public school system that leaves much to be desired when it comes to sex education and consequently does little to offset the sexual content our young people are exposed to. It could even be argued that the school system sometimes contributes to the problem by not doing enough to minimize sexual behaviors that occur in schools. Our community-based organizations, some of which actually do offer some effective sex education programs, do not reach enough of an audience, and our religious institutions for the most part do not offer sex education on a scale that could have any impact. So that leaves us parents to provide sex education to our children. As I said previously, of all the possible influential sources of sexual guidance for young people, we the parents can have the greatest impact on our children's sexual behavior. You could stack up all the sex education programs that do exist and none of them would be as successful as the parents who have established themselves as approachable by their children on sexual matters. In an ideal world, the schools would use an empirically validated sex education program and work collaboratively with parents who are approachable and who communicate effectively with their children. But until we can get the school sex education programs in order, the one thing we parents have control over is our ability to be the number one influence in our child's sexual lives. You can do it—and this book will show you the way. Read on.

CHAPTER 2

Helping Our Children Make Sense of the Sexualized Wall

I will have much to say throughout this book on how we as parents can assist our children in making sense of the wall of sexualized messages, how we can be approachable, and what to say to our kids when various situations arise. First, let's take a preliminary look at how we can help our kids manage and negotiate their wall, and how we might be able to mitigate some of the more deleterious effects of the wall.

We Can't Run Away from the Wall

For all the concern that I am raising about the hypersexualization of children today, by no means do I think that we are seeing the beginning of the end or that we are facing some sort of Armageddon concerning the future of sexual behavior in America. We certainly have the capacity to assist our children through these highly sexualized times and many parents and adults are doing just that. But unfortunately we can expect to shelter our kids only so much from their exposure to sexualized matters. We can't expect them to be able to avoid or escape their walls of sexualized messages. I speak to many parents who want to try to cover their children's eyes and ears, believing that somehow their kids will be able to avoid the wall. To be sure, we should all try to minimize our children's exposure to damaging sexualized messages. However, we can't expect to constantly shield them from those realities that exist in the world. We have to accept that our kids will have some exposure. So we need to be there for them on a regular and ongoing basis, prepared to counter and buffer the many confusing messages they receive from their sexualized wall and to help them make sense of what they are exposed to.

By doing this, we can expect to add our own helpful blocks to our child's wall of sex information. Remember that not all of our child's sexualized wall has to be problematic, confusing, or harmful. As parents, we add our own blocks to our child's wall and if we communicate effectively and smartly, those blocks will help promote a healthy and positive sexuality in our child and actually counter those blocks that are less than desirable. When we tell our child why we love them so much, and then go on to give them accurate information about sex and sexuality, provide fair and consistent boundaries for how they should behave sexually, and offer them guidance regarding how to better understand the sexual messages they do receive, we add positive sexual messages to their sexualized wall—and counter the damaging messages.

Preparing to Counter the Wall

I have five key points for you as you begin your effort to counteract the potentially damaging sexual messages your child is receiving:

- Recognize and accept the fact that your child is being affected by these messages.

- Do not wait for your child to ask questions about sex before talking about such matters.
- Take advantage of teachable moments.
- Stay on top of what your child is experiencing and be vigilant in monitoring his or her life and world.
- Reflect on your parenting style.

Let's look at each of these in turn.

Face the Facts

First and foremost, you must recognize and accept the fact that your child is being affected by potentially damaging sexual messages. I have spoken to far too many parents who think their children somehow remain innocent when it comes to sex and sexuality: "Oh, my ten-year-old son is so naive. He doesn't have a clue about sex, or any interest in it, for that matter. I don't even think he knows what sex is."

Yeah, right, and what planet do you live on? I say to myself. By thinking this way, parents only postpone the inevitable conclusion that we underestimate what our kids are doing, what they think about, and what they know. There's a considerable body of research now that confirms this.[1] I suppose it's only natural for us to want to believe that our kids don't do all those bad things that other kids do. But we would be wise to rethink our assumptions about what our kids do and don't do sexually.

So parents, let's all face up to it right now. Our kids are sexual human beings, they think about sex, they've heard and seen their fair share of sexual matters, and they have many things around them that will promote their interest in sex. Of course, this will all depend to some degree on their age. All things considered, the ten-year-old will have more information than the seven-year-old, and the seven-year-old will have more than the four- or five-year-old. Nevertheless, even your charming and cute four- or five-year-old will be well on her way to various sexual exposures as she begins kindergarten. Put twenty five-year-olds together for any length of time and you will see a variety of behaviors and abilities—as well as different levels of sexual curiosity. They will express that curiosity, and at some point your little one will express hers. Most of the behaviors will range from curiosity regarding the differences in girls' and boys' body parts (the oldie but goodie "playing doctor"), occasional boyfriend-girlfriend role-play, pretend kissing, some silly talk about things like "wee-wee" and "tush," some peeking at others in the bathroom or bedroom, and of course masturbation. But, as I've been saying, far too frequently we now hear and see things from five-year-olds that we hardly ever heard or saw before.

Even though five-year-olds are quite innocent and fairly oblivious to sexual matters, sexualized behavior in five-year-olds is emerging far too frequently. We now see kids this young touching others' genitals; we hear them say things like "I want to sex you"; we see them use force and coercion to get others to disrobe, touch each other, and lie on top of each other; and we even know of some who perform oral sex. I'll have much more to say on this later, but I also want to bring this to your attention early on, because if you're a parent of a little one you absolutely need to heed the sex contamination factor at these young ages.

The important thing here is not to be naive about your child's sexualized wall of messages. For if you are, you will fail to appreciate just how much your child needs you to be approachable on sexual matters. Should you fall prey to thinking that your son or daughter is entirely innocent, you will pay the price for not paying attention. Your child is going to be exposed to—and affected by—sexual messages and behavior much earlier than you think.

FROM THE MOUTHS OF BABES

A parent once told me that her little boy's kindergarten teacher had called her and reported that, after being told by one of the girls in his class that she had a boyfriend, the little boy promptly asked her if she had had sex with him yet. Needless to say, the little girl's mom was upset. None of this is especially problematic, but it does represent how things have changed over the years.

How should a parent respond to this type of behavior? You could say to the little girl, "Oh, Tommy was being silly, and he shouldn't have said what he said." Be prepared to clarify what sex means if she appears to want to take your conversation further (see page 101). But if she's satisfied with your response, let it go for now.

The boy is another matter. Since he's the one who used the word *sex*, you could say to him, "Do you know what sex is?" Chances are he would say it means kissing or that he doesn't know, and you could say, "Well, let me tell you what it means. Sex is much more than kissing or hugging. It's something that only adults who love each other do, like mommy and daddy. What happens is that mom and dad take their clothes off and lie in bed next to each other and start to hold and kiss each other." I think that at this point the boy would probably not want to hear you say anything more. He'd probably cover his ears and say something like, "Yuck, that's disgusting," and that would be it. You see, five-year-olds really don't want to hear too much about sex, but this little guy needs to understand that what he said can mean a whole lot more than what he thought it did.

Don't Delay!

Do not wait for your child to ask questions about sex before speaking to her about such matters. She may never ask you those questions. You must be one or two steps ahead of your child, knowing from a developmental standpoint what your child needs to know about sex and sexuality. You've made an excellent decision by picking up this book and, by the time you're done, you'll know exactly what your child needs to know and at what age they need to know it. This book will also help you better understand parenting issues and parenting styles that pertain to our role as sex educators (see later in this chapter and chapter 9). None of us went to school to learn how to be good parents, yet it is without question the hardest thing we will ever do in life.

Take Advantage of Teachable Moments

If you and your child are watching television, listening to music, or passing by a billboard that is sending a sexualized message, be ready to intervene and help your child make sense of it. Don't be shy. Share with your kid what you think about the sexual message. Share your thoughts, your beliefs, and your values—whatever you feel would be helpful for your child.

I will elaborate much more on such teachable moments later on. These are the major way in which we provide most of our sexuality education and guidance to our children. For now, suffice it to say that we need to learn how to recognize teachable moments. Many of us think that we have to have those formal sit-down talks with our kids when we communicate about sex and sexuality. I personally recommend them, but it's actually in spontaneous real-life situations that we provide most of our guidance about sex and sexuality to our kids. For example, perhaps you've caught your seven-year-old masturbating on the couch in the living room: "Hey, sweetheart, I know it feels good to masturbate but as

I've told you before it's a private behavior and I really don't want to have to see you do it. You can go up to your bedroom for that." You acknowledge the behavior, you share your values (in this case, you support the behavior), and you put it in context with boundaries (it's a private behavior for the bedroom).

Or you're walking your eight-year-old daughter to school in an urban area and you pass an adult sex shop with a strap-on dildo and a naked blow-up doll in the window. Your kid looks at it with confusion, and your first instinct is to pick up your walking pace and hope you can get away without having to say anything. What the heck do you say to an eight-year-old about dildos and blow-up rubber dolls? Well, being the good parent that you are, you realize that you need to do the right thing and address with her what she's just seen. You can't do what so many adults do—that is, engage in the age-old parental practice of avoidance response. I hear so many stories of parents avoiding uncomfortable situations involving their child, in the hopes that they will just go away. Well, they don't go away; they only come back to haunt you. Don't let her add these images to her sexualized wall and allow them to affect her as they may without any adult intervention. Intervene now: "Well, honey, there was some pretty weird stuff there in that shop window, huh?" Wait a second to see how she responds. I'm not sure if an eight-year-old would notice the dildo or not, but let's assume that she does. "Yeah, why was there a naked doll and fake penis in that store?" she asks. Your response might be something like this: "You know, as crazy as it sounds, there are some adults who buy things like fake penises and naked dolls. I know it sounds nuts, but it's true. Some adults think it's kind of funny to do that; they do it as a joke. But there are some adults who use them as though they were real by touching and holding them. Daddy (or Mommy) and I think that's silly, but if some adults want them, I don't think they'll cause any harm."

You don't need to worry about your eight-year-old being negatively affected by saying this to her. She probably doesn't have much interest in any of it to begin with. But I do think you need to address the fact that she has seen these things. She may well see them again, perhaps numerous times, if she goes to school down the block from the shop. At some point she may begin to talk with her peers about what she has seen and things could really start to get a little out of hand if she doesn't have a context in which to place the information. Help your child process the many confusing messages that are out there. By intervening early and giving some context to what she sees, it is likely that your thoughts on the matter will stick with her and mitigate future exposures to the adult shop.

Pay Attention

You need to be aware of what your child is experiencing. Be vigilant in monitoring his life and world. This applies to parenting in general, of course, but it is especially true as it pertains to sex and sexuality.

Know who your child's peers and friends are and who *their* parents are. Many parents don't. You have to find out some of the values that your child's friends espouse. This will give you a window of insight into their thoughts on sexual matters. Plus, it's just a good thing to do on many levels. You might as well start early on this, as you're going to really need to key in on his peer group when he's eleven to fourteen years of age—a critical time for peer group formation—so start practicing now.

If you have computers in your house make sure your ten-, eleven-, or twelve-year-old does not have unsupervised access to them. Make sure your kids don't sign on to Facebook, MySpace, or any other social networking site.

Of course, you know you will be challenged. "But why, Mom?" your daughter asks. "My friends are allowed to join."

"Because I love you, plain and simple, and you are too young for this kind of virtual interaction. Plus you are a unique individual—you are not your friends—and you will be better off without it."

Just take a firm stand, especially with your younger children. Some of your kids will protest, shout, and kick like crazy when you tell them no, but that's just too bad. Tell them that you will *not* let them be on the Internet without supervision, and you will not let them join a social network. In fact, parents of teenagers thirteen, fourteen, and fifteen years of age should do the same—certainly with regard to social networking.

Monitor your children's relationships with each other. If your kids are three or four years apart, for example, make sure you know what the older one is teaching or possibly showing the younger one. Do not assume that just because they're siblings the older one won't corrupt or hurt the younger one. I had a parent tell me once that her eight-year-old son bathes with her five-year-old and when they're in there he pokes and pinches the little one's penis and butt. She asked me whether or not she should allow them to continue bathing. My message to her was very simple; it is never a good idea to allow siblings of significantly different ages to bathe together. Don't believe me? Then go ahead and allow it, but please keep an eye on them. If you don't have time to supervise, *don't let them bathe together.*

Make sure you have parental controls on the television set if your child has one in her bedroom. Even with the controls, check periodically that your child hasn't cracked the codes. Our kids always seem to stay a step or two ahead of us in the realm of technology. In fact, we should take little for granted when it comes to our kids. They're wonderful and lovely, and we can trust them—that is, to a point. You should always keep in mind that your child has the potential to do things you would not want her to do. Keep your eyes and ears open at all times, and try to develop the ability to "see from the back of your head." I was asked recently by a parent of a fifth grader whether or not I think it's a good idea for her to snoop on her child. My instant answer: "Of course you should." Actually, what some call *snooping* I call proactive monitoring, and it is an essential ingredient to effective parenting. Naturally, you want to give your children increasing opportunities for independence as they demonstrate they are capable and responsible enough to handle things. But make no mistake about it, you are in charge and you will proactively monitor their lives as long as you feel it is necessary to do so. And you should do this especially with regard to sexual matters.

Reflect on Your Parenting Style

There's a ton of research out there on parenting styles and we know a lot about what style of parenting works well and what doesn't. When you sift through the research, you'll find basically four styles of parenting:

- *Authoritarian* parents have very rigid rules ("My way or the highway") and frequently rely on punishment to shape behavior.

- *Permissive* parents avoid confrontation or argument; they want to be friends with their kids.

- *Uninvolved* parents, as the term implies, provide for basic needs but stay pretty much on the sidelines when it comes to their children.

- *Authoritative* parents are, as you may deduce, the ones who find balance, have clearly articulated boundaries of what is right and wrong, allow for views to be shared, and use positive reinforcement to shape behavior. This is the kind of parent you want to be.[2]

I won't focus in any great detail on parenting styles, but I will touch on the ingredients of the various styles in terms of the role of an approachable parent on sexual matters, with a greater emphasis on the authoritative style. You should educate yourself on the merits of authoritative parenting and make every effort to practice its effective components.

CAUGHT IN THE SOCIAL NETWORK

My boss recently confided in me that his twelve-year-old daughter was being exposed to sexual talk on her social networking page from a male peer who wanted to kiss and lick virtually every private part of one of her female friends. His daughter was very upset the day this happened—she eventually told her mother, who then shared the news with my boss. When I told my boss that he needed to help her process what she had experienced and then close her social networking account, he became conflicted over whether or not he should do that. He believed his daughter would protest vehemently and he wasn't sure if he wanted to have that confrontation with her.

Ah, not wanting a confrontation! He's exhibiting the classic wishy-washy response of a permissive parent (which I will address in more detail later). What he should be doing is to be empathetic but take a firm stand with his daughter. He should say to her, "Honey, what have you learned from this experience?" He should let her respond—but the message he wants her to get and needs to steer her toward is that it takes a lot to really get to know the core of an individual. And even then you still can't be absolutely certain what the person might or might not do. Then he should follow up by saying, "I can imagine how shocked you are. I am really glad that you shared this with me. I think this boy was way out of line. What he did was wrong and he should apologize." Finally, he needs to tell her that she must close her page on her social networking site. There's no magical statement to make for this one. The bottom line is that she's too young for any of this, and as her father it's his job to protect his daughter.

Being Authentic in Our Approach to Challenging the Wall

To enhance your chances that you will be approachable and the most influential source of sexual guidance for your child, *be authentic* when teaching your child about sex and sexuality. We are all sex educators. The mere fact that we are parents dictates this, and—just like the teachers I train to teach sex education—we need to be authentic when we go about our instruction with our kids. This means we need to take our kids to a real place when we teach them.

Look Both Ways Before Crossing

Think about how you taught (or will teach) your child to cross the street safely. That is, you will have endless conversations about crossing at the corner, looking both ways before venturing out into the street, and crossing on the green. You'll role-play different situations that she could encounter when crossing a street, creating scenarios that could actually happen. For example, a driver might run a red light, or she might come to a large intersection where multiple cars want to turn simultaneously, or an intersection with no lights and only stop signs; you will create every imaginable situation that your child could possibly encounter when crossing the street. And of course you will take her out to the street and actually practice crossing it correctly and in a way that reduces the risk of accident. When you do, you will be doing *authentic instruction* (see sidebar) in its purest form: teaching your child by having her actually practice the very thing that you want her to learn.

AUTHENTIC INSTRUCTION

Authentic instruction, or *authentic teaching*, is a form of instruction that uses circumstances that are as close to real life as possible. In its purest form, authentic instruction involves learning by actually doing. If you are teaching about climbing a rock wall, you have your pupil practice climbing a rock wall. Or if you are teaching your child to cross the street, you actually practice crossing a street with him. Admittedly, it is harder to use real-life experiences when teaching your child about sexuality (you can't have your child actually have sex, can you?). But there are many strategies that come close to creating a sense of real-life circumstances that you can use. Throughout the book, I will give you examples of authentic instruction strategies for the issues we're covering—issues like sexual feelings, peer pressure, sexual decision making, and being male and female. I will offer some strategies for addressing love, respect, and trust in chapter 3.

Imagine a Real-Life Scenario

When you are teaching your child about sex and sexuality, come as close as you possibly can to having him experience what it is you want him to learn. So, for example, if you want your ten-year-old to understand how to avoid sexual peer pressure, you might create a scenario where he is older and in middle school and that drop-dead gorgeous girl comes on to him when at a party at a friend's house:

"What are you going to do when she tells you you're hot, touches your butt, and wants you to come with her and her friends to another party at someone else's house?" you ask him. "You feel so flattered she's noticed you and no one else, your heart is jumping out of your chest, you've got butterflies in your stomach, and your pulse is racing. You are even getting an erection. So, what are you going to do?"

He will likely say he doesn't know (he's still only ten). So you will guide him through various options for managing this dilemma and then cap it off with what you hope he will do, which is of course to avoid any sexual contact. You'll remind him that all feelings are normal but that ultimately he needs to make a choice that reduces the risk for sexual involvement.

Going through this scenario with your ten-year-old child is a perfect example of how you can approach the concept that "ten is the new sixteen." It's hard for a ten-year-old to fully relate to this scenario, simply because kids of this age are not likely to encounter a peer pressure situation like this. But you want to start to get your ten-year-old to think about these sorts of situations now rather than when they are thirteen or fourteen. Remember, it is much easier to reinforce the concept of sexual abstinence with kids who have little or no interest in actually having sex, rather than trying to do it at a later age when interest is on the rise.

Let's look at another example of authentic teaching. Your six-year-old comes to you complaining about a boy in her class who has on several occasions tried to touch her buttocks and between her legs. He has also tried to do this with some of the other kids in her class. Tell her she did the right thing to tell you, and that she should always tell the teacher when he even tries to touch her. Tell her you will address this with the teacher and the principal, and that they will all work together to keep him from trying this behavior in the future. You tell her that some kids have trouble keeping their hands to themselves, and that they will do this to either get attention or make themselves feel bigger and better than the other kids. Then, say: "Next time he tries to do this to you, tell him 'no' in a very firm voice and go and tell your teacher. When he wants to work with you or play a game with you, you can tell him you will but that you will not allow him to touch you."

You and your daughter can role-play different situations when the boy is being appropriate in his interactions with her and other times when he tries to touch. Each time, have your daughter act out how she would handle each situation. Role-play is an authentic technique for teaching about sex and sexuality.

Share Your Values About Life and Sexuality

Always share your particular values about whatever you are trying to teach. Values drive our sense of what is right, what is wrong, what is to be cherished, and what is to be avoided. Your children need your guidance and instruction in order to form their own value systems as they develop.

For example, let's say you want to address the topic of HIV/AIDS with your five-year-old. A values-related issue that will come up is the acceptance and kind treatment of persons with HIV/AIDS, or for that matter anyone who has a potentially life-threatening illness. You will want to instill in your young child the value of helping those who are sick and ill.

Or perhaps you want to discuss homosexuality with your five-year-old. This is a perfect time to help your child develop what will be a life-long acceptance and tolerance of persons who are gay and lesbian. (If you do not adhere to this view that all people are to be accepted regardless of their sexuality, then shame on you! People are attacked and killed in this country every year just because they are thought to be gay or lesbian, so enough of this thinking once and for all.) Discussing tolerance in general only strengthens a young person's ability to do just that—become tolerant. Discussing homosexuality with your five-year-old child will not cause him or her to become gay, just as discussing tolerance of persons of a different color will not change your child's skin tone.

So how do you explain homosexuality to your child in a respectful, nonjudgmental way? You start with something like, "You know, just like men and women can fall in love with each other, so can two men or two women. Two men who fall in love with each other are called gay men. Two women who do so are called lesbian women. They are also called homosexual." It's likely that at this point your five-year-old will be pretty bored and say "Okay" and be done with it. You could then follow up by saying, "There are some people who disapprove of people who are gay and lesbian. Sometimes people try to hurt people who are gay or lesbian. I think that is so terrible and wrong. I want you to grow up with respect for people who are homosexual." And keep in mind that it's entirely possible your five-year-old may actually be homosexual him- or herself—which is one more reason why it's so important to reinforce values of acceptance and kindness. You want your child to accept him- or herself regardless of sexual orientation.

Helping to shape and instill values in your child is no small matter. Your child's sexualized wall will have many messages that reflect various values about sex and sexuality. And of course many of them will be values that you would not want your child to develop and ones you will need to counter: messages that glorify the objectification and denigration of women, messages that tell young males that the more women you can have sex with the better man you'll be, messages that damage a young person's body image, messages that promote sexual irresponsibility, and a whole bunch of other messages that will run contrary to the values you want to instill in your kid.

Let Your Kid Know What You Think Is Right and Wrong

When you share your values about sex and sexuality with your kids, you are also letting them know what you think is right and wrong. You can't do better as a parent or do more to add to your approachability than when you share with your child the boundaries you expect for their sexual behavior and positively reinforce those boundaries on a consistent basis. You're doing this when you take the following kinds of actions:

- You say to your ten-year-old fifth grader, "I really don't think you're old enough to have a boyfriend yet," and then follow that up some time later with "I am pleased that you haven't had a boyfriend yet."

- You tell your eight-year-old, "When you say, 'That's so gay,' it really troubles me because I think it's insulting to homosexuals," and then follow up several days later with "I've noticed that lately you haven't used the word *gay* in that way that bothers me. I'm very proud of you."

- You tell your six-year-old, who may have had a habit of touching himself in public areas of your home, "It's okay to touch your penis and masturbate, but it's a private behavior," and you follow the next week with, "You know, you haven't masturbated in the living room lately and Mommy is very proud of you."

- You tell your ten-year-old, "I do not believe anyone should have sex until they are an adult and in love," and in the following years you periodically tell her, "You consistently impress me with your decision to wait to have intercourse until adulthood. I love you very much."

Our children need to hear from us what we believe to be right and wrong behavior when it comes to sexual matters. Why are too many of us reluctant to do this? So many parents who come to my school presentations don't want to commit to drawing the line with their kids on different sexual behaviors. Some have actually told me they had sex before they were an adult and it didn't ruin their lives. "So why be so harsh on our kids?" one mother asked me. A dad recently said, "I should tell my daughter she can't have sex before being in love? Why? I didn't."

It is our job as parents to set limits. We just have to set those limits and talk about them in ways that allow our kids to listen to us. And we can't wait for their middle school years to do this! We estimate that 7 percent to 10 percent of kids in the United States will have intercourse before thirteen years of age. That's between five million and seven and a half million kids who will have intercourse before becoming a teenager.[3]

So you say to your eight-, nine-, or ten-year-old, "I love you, and because I love you I hope that you don't have sex until you are an adult, and then, only with someone you respect, trust, and love." If your daughter or son acts as though she or he can't stand to hear you say that—because, after all, this is still pretty young—you can say, "Okay, okay, I understand this is tough to hear, but trust me, it's really important that you understand what your parents think about the right time to have sex. And it's better to hear this now than when you are older and maybe it's too late. We will continue to have talks like this with you as you grow older." Many high school kids have told me, "Hey, Dr. Fred, when you told us that stuff in fifth grade I didn't think it was that important, but I sure do now."

Our kids need to know where we stand and what we think is right and wrong about sexual matters: masturbation, homosexuality, contraception, abortion, oral sex, sex toys, skirt length, pants hanging below the underwear line, and on and on. Our kids will at some point develop their own values for these issues and it is essential that we share with them what ours are before they form their own. You can't be shy about any of this stuff. Let's say, for instance, you believe the following:

- Masturbation is fine but private.
- Gays and lesbians should never be discriminated against or denigrated.

- Condoms are the only form of *contraception* that is effective against HIV, but abstinence is the most effective choice against HIV.
- Abortion is horrible but needs to be legal.
- Oral sex is fine for adults in loving, committed relationships, but you can get HIV and other diseases if you engage in it—and oral sex *is* sex.
- If a girl dresses in a sexy way, heterosexual boys will think she wants to do it (and they will want to do it).

These are values statements, and you can share them with your child by ten years of age. So where do *you* stand on the issues? What are *your* values? We will explore many as we go through this book together.

Form a Bond

I probably cannot say too much about bonding. It is perhaps the single most important factor in a child's life—forming a loving, respectful, trusting relationship over time with a significant adult. And who better to fill that role than Mom or Dad or another designated guardian? So much of what I have been talking about here in this chapter lends itself to helping us bond with our child. Bonding with our kids means so much more than being friends with them, or doing things with them, or "hanging" with them, or having them do as we ask. Bonding is a meaningful and deep, insightful, everlasting, symbiotic relationship with another human being—in this case with your child.

Bonding with your child will create a protective barrier that will insulate him against some of the most significant risk factors facing young people today.[4] If you bond with your child, the chances that your child will engage in drug use, commit a violent act, or engage in some form of risky sexual behavior will decrease. That's right: if you make it your business to bond with your children, you will increase the odds that your child will avoid these destructive behaviors. So much of this goes back to what I was saying earlier. We hold such significant power to positively shape our children's sexual behavior.

What does bonding mean?

- Sharing your values about sex and setting limits on your child's sexual behavior
- Acting authoritatively by reinforcing the positive behavior your child engages in rather than punishing the negative
- Communicating sexual information so your child knows that being a sexual being can be enriching and life enhancing if she makes responsible decisions
- Telling your child you love him—and why you do
- Monitoring your child's sexualized wall and intervening as needed to mitigate the negative and harmful sexual messages

A Pause to Reflect

Before we move on to considering what's at stake in our efforts to ensure a healthy, happy sexual future for our children, please take some time to think about the following points:

- Sex and sexuality can be fantastic and life enhancing; they can also be horrific and deadly.
- Your child desperately needs you to be involved in her or his sexual growth and development. You need to believe this 100 percent and be on board with it without question from this moment on.

- Your children are sexual beings and will be until death. How will they express their femaleness or maleness? You need to think about penises, breasts, vaginas, short skirts, revealing blouses, low-hanging pants that show underwear, abortion, pregnancy, doing it (when, with whom), masturbation, homo-sexuality, bisexuality, femininity, masculinity, kissing, tongue kissing, dildos, vibrators, sexual harassment, online chatting and networking, dating, getting felt up, hand jobs, anal intercourse, three-ways, S&M, nudity, and on and on. Will you address all this with your children, and, if so, when?

- What, in your view, is sexually right and what is sexually wrong? And how will these views and values affect your children's sexuality?

- What sort of man do you want your son to be? What sort of woman do you want your daughter to be?

The answers to these questions are critical, because there is so much at stake. We will take a closer look at what's on the line in chapter 4. But first we're going to focus on what I call *the big three*: love, respect, and trust. They are *the* most important factors for achieving a happy, healthy, fulfilling sexuality—and, for that matter, a happy, healthy, fulfilling life.

CHAPTER 3

The Three Biggest Sex Words in this Book: Love, Respect, and Trust

This is the most important part of the book. The message is simple, although it can be hard to put it into practice: *you should only have sexual intercourse with someone with whom you share mutual love, respect, and trust.* I know some if not many readers will think I am naive, but it is a message we lost somewhere over the years on our way to sexual enlightenment in this country. Sexual pleasure has taken precedence over anything remotely resembling emotional connectedness, and our children are the biggest losers. I am disheartened when I speak to teenagers who not only struggle to understand how to identify when one has found true love, respect, and trust, but who also do not necessarily believe that one must have these in a relationship prior to engaging in sexual intercourse. It is very likely that their parents have not had significant or meaningful discussions with them about the importance of these three ingredients.

Am I right? Can you tell me how much time you have spent with your child addressing what I call the "big three"? Have you helped your child learn how to recognize love, respect, and trust? Whether your kid is five, ten, or fifteen years of age, have you done your best to instill in her the importance of forging a relationship with your life partner that is steeped in mutual love, respect, and trust? If we want our children to value being responsible, to show respect for others, to be trustworthy and honest, and to have empathy toward others, it follows that we would want them to seek these values when it comes to deciding whom to share sexual intercourse with.

The Power of the Big Three

It is important to share with your children, as early as you can, that having these three ingredients in a relationship will reduce the risk of sexual harm (such as date rape), sexually transmitted disease, unwanted pregnancy, and other nasty consequences of physical intimacy. When you have absolute mutual respect and trust with someone, and you share real love with that person, you never have to worry that he or she will ever deliberately try to hurt you, cheat you, or dishonor you. This is important stuff—consider how many people will sexually abuse others during their relationship, lie about their HIV status or STDs, be irresponsible and not wear a condom during sex, cheat on their partner, and in general treat their partner like crap. But when you really have love, respect, and trust, those negative things will not happen.

I have met many, many parents during my presentations who believe these three core values are what they want for their child. They want their kids to grow up to be responsible adults. They want their kids to have and show respect for others, to be trustworthy, honest, and empathetic. They also want them to forge relationships with people who share the same core values, with the hope and expectation that their children will be treated as they would treat others. Yet when I ask them whether they would want their children to be sexually active only when they have real love, respect, and trust in a relationship, many of them say that this would be expecting too much and would be far too unrealistic. "After all," many of them say, "what's wrong with just enjoying a good sexual relationship?"

Are you wondering the exact same thing? *What's the big deal about two people wanting to share sex together?* Why do we have to tell our kids that they can't have sex, can't do something that can be fun as hell to do, unless they are in love first and have mutual respect and trust with the person they're going to be doing it with? "If *I* didn't live by those standards," parents have asked me, "then why should I ask my kids to do it? Plus it's so old-fashioned." There are parents who believe I go too far when I tell them to use my standard of love, respect, and trust when teaching their child to identify the right time for sex.

But let's look at reality. When someone truly loves you and has unmistakable respect for you, and is someone you can trust, would you worry that this person might deliberately try to hurt you? That this person might knowingly give you a sexually transmitted infection or HIV? That this person might just be using you for sexual purposes? That this person would leave you high and dry if you were to become pregnant? Or that this person would try to take advantage of you sexually—force you to have sex when you did not want it, for example? The answer in every case is no. Think about it. If we all waited to have sexual intercourse until we had true love, respect, and trust, we would be able to minimize many of the health-related problems that are the result of sexual risk behaviors. Unwanted pregnancies, sexually transmitted infections including HIV, and sexual assault would all be reduced. Sadly, however, for the past several decades we have struggled as a society to get control of these major health risk problems among young people. In fact, sexual risk behaviors among young people now represent one of the six major causes of morbidity and mortality in the United States.

Now, let's forget the sex stuff for a minute. For any relationship to survive and thrive, think about how essential the big three are. Think how crucial our message is when we explore with our kids how true love, respect, and trust establish a bond between two people that is not easily broken. Physical appearance, material comforts and money, good sex, enjoying the same music, and all the other things that play a part in a relationship really do pale next to developing respect and trust. Put them together with true love, which can only come from mutually congruent values, a sense of empathy for another, and goodness of heart, and they collectively make for the deepest of connections with another person. Of course, conflicts will arise in any committed, loving relationship, but when love, respect, and trust are present, those conflicts are easier to resolve.

Along the way, we will also impart valuable insight regarding decision making and critical thinking about sexual behavior with our kids, the value of contraception and most importantly condom use, and guidance on how to evaluate and manage interpersonal experiences. In short, we will prepare them for as many real-life occurrences as possible so that when they become adults, if they at times engage in sexual behavior with others without the big three ingredients, they'll do so in ways that dramatically reduce their risks.

Send the Message Early and Often

When you tell your five-year-old that a baby is made when a sperm cell joins together with an egg cell (see chapter 6), you also need to begin your discussion with the statement that this should only happen when two people love each other. Even if you have yet to mention sexual intercourse, you need to discuss making a baby in the context of love between two people: "You know, sweetheart, two people should only have a baby if they are in love with each other. When two people are in love it means that they would never deliberately do anything to one another that is hurtful or bad." Along with the message of love should also come some mention of respect and trust. It is not too early for your five-year-old to begin to learn what these traits are and how they relate to child bearing: "When two people love each other it also means they have respect for each other. This means that they each believe that the other person always wants to do what is right and good, and they like that about each other. It also means that they can trust each other. When two people trust each other, they never have to worry that one of them might do anything to hurt the other or do something to make them feel bad. It's so important that two people who want to have a baby love, respect, and trust each other very much."

When your child is eight and you have your first conversation about sexual intercourse (see chapters 6 and 8), you want to make sure that you reinforce how important these qualities are in a relationship: "You know how we have spoken about how important it is that two people who want to have a baby should love, respect, and trust each other? Well, I want you to know that I feel the same way regarding having sex. When people love each other they always have the other person's best interests at heart. When they respect each other they never have to worry that one of them would make the other have sex when he didn't want to. When they trust each other they never have to worry that one of them would cheat by having sex with someone else, or worry that the other has a sexually transmitted infection. They would never have to worry that one of them would just use the other for sex."

Try to highlight real-life examples of love, respect, and trust for your children (we'll talk more about this later). When I speak to students, for example, I tell them that although I have been married for thirty-five years I still cannot say with 100 percent certainty that my wife will never cheat me, hurt me, or deliberately try to disappoint me. No one can predict with absolute certainty what another person will or will not do. However, I can come pretty close to being able to do it when it comes to my wife. As I look back over the nearly forty years that I've known her I have never caught her trying to do anything that would hurt me. So I can with some accuracy predict that she will never do so in the future. I tell my students that the same principle applies to them: the longer they know someone, the more accurately they can judge whether they can trust that person.

When your child is nine or ten years old and you have already discussed sexual intercourse and oral and anal sex with her (see chapter 8), you should still be mindful of the importance of highlighting the three biggest sex words in this book. You could say something like the following:

"Can you believe that a lot of people who have HIV in their bodies, and know that they have it, do not disclose that information to the person or persons they have sex with?[1] It is amazing to me that there are people who know that they have HIV and yet do not tell the people that they have sex with. As you think about this fact, what one really important thing does this tells you?"

Your daughter may look up at you and just shrug her shoulders.

"Really. I can't believe people would do that, but unfortunately there are many who do. What does this tell you about a lot of people who have sex?"

"I guess it means that there are people who don't care a whole lot about the people they have sex with," your daughter replies.

"Bingo! That's got to be it," you say to her. "If they really did care about them, they would tell the people they have sex with that they have the virus. Think about it. If you loved someone, you would certainly be honest about having a virus that is transmitted through sexual intercourse before having sexual intercourse with that person. That is just a given if you really loved the person; you would never want to hurt him. But I guess if you didn't love the person, you wouldn't bother to share this information with him. Do you see just how important love is when it comes to having sexual intercourse?"

WHAT PASSES FOR LOVE

Many teens don't understand what true love is. Countless times I have had teenagers tell me, "Oh, Dr. Fred, I love him and he loves me. He'll always love me, he'll never leave me, and he'll never hurt me. Our love is forever." But after a little questioning I find out that they've known the other person for a grand total of five, six, or seven months.

So I say to them, "Well, I'll tell you one thing, if you become pregnant he's probably going to leave you."

"What, Dr. Fred?" they reply. "Are you kidding me? He would never leave me if I was pregnant."

"Sure, he would," I reply. "There are many, many guys who get their girlfriends pregnant who leave the relationship. They don't stick around and take responsibility and that's a fact!"

When I made these statements to a class of eighth graders, one of the boys vehemently protested, saying, "That sure wouldn't be me, Dr. Fred!"

"Well," I said, "you would have to prove me wrong, then, because the odds are very much against you. The truth of the matter is that many boys leave their girlfriends high and dry and it's often because they really didn't love them."

Other factors that cause teen boys to leave their pregnant girlfriends include immaturity, fear, and the fact that they are just kids, of course. All of this is why we want to actively encourage our kids to delay intercourse until they are older, in love, and in a better position to behave responsibly. If you follow my advice in this book, you'll have a far better chance of having this happen for your children.

Is This Love?

From a developmental standpoint it does take a certain amount of emotional intelligence and maturity to fully appreciate what true love is and to know when you've found it. It is one of the major reasons why teenagers (and perhaps many adults as well) need a major course in "Love 101." We really don't invest a lot of time or energy teaching our children how to recognize love. Consequently, many of our adolescents will have relationships where they are certain they are in love only to find out, often the hard way, that they weren't really in love at all. So we need to make a concerted effort to teach our children what love is and how to recognize it when it actually happens.

Oh, there's plenty of passion out there and a lot of emotions that masquerade as love. Many people have experienced the feelings, emotions, and attitudes initially associated with love in a relationship, only to find that they were insufficient to make for an enduring and lasting love. That is, what we thought at first must have been love was really only a sort of passion, infatuation, or lust. Rings a bell, doesn't it? You can probably remember a time or two when you thought you were very much in love, only to find out as time went by that it wasn't true love at all. You may have acted upon those feelings in ways that, in retrospect, were not in your best interests. Even as adults many people have a whole lot of difficulty knowing when they have found real love, so we can only imagine how tough it must be for young people.

Our kids have a much more difficult job of navigating the love issue than many of us did, and far more so than our parents and grandparents. This is because they live in a culture where many more teenagers and young adults are sexually active. And when a relationship goes bad, it's considerably more complicated when sex has been involved than when things haven't gone that far. Consequently, the misidentification of love among young people today has far greater consequences than it did when many of us were growing up. Today, a kid may think she's in love and move much closer to having intimate sexual situations than she would have in past generations. And the closer one gets to a mutual sex encounter, the closer one gets to experience a sexual risk situation: pregnancy, sexually transmitted infection, sexual assault, and so on. Because of this, a major part of our job as parents must be to help our kids appreciate how difficult it is to know when you have true love with someone, and to develop a skill set that allows them to differentiate true love from something that passes for it. I hope you can see how important it is to focus much of your attention on identifying love in your efforts to be approachable for your kids. Love should form the foundation of the many messages about sexuality that we will want to impart to our children as they grow and develop.

A True Friend

I give a lot of talks about friendship with kids at different grade levels as part of a broader conversation about sexuality. When I tell fourth- and fifth-grade kids about my trust in my wife after all these years, I follow it by asking them about their friends. I think that a very useful way to help kids understand love is to ask them to consider the difference between their regular friends and best friends. The discussion goes something like this:

"How many of you have had a friend whom you are no longer close to because he or she did something you didn't like?" Just about every hand in the class goes up. "So give me some examples of what your so-called 'friend' did that made you break off the friendship with her or him?"

One kid says, "Well, my friend lied to me one time." Another student says, "My friend stole five dollars from me; I couldn't believe it." And yet another says, "Mine blamed me for something bad that she did and I was the one who got in trouble for it."

Next, I ask, "How many of you have a best friend?" Virtually every hand goes up. "And what makes a best friend different from just an ordinary or regular friend?"

Various answers are given by the students, but they are very certain that there is a major difference. "They're much nicer than just regular friends, Dr. Fred," says one. "You know your best friend much longer and much better than just regular friends," says another. "They are always there for you, and you can always rely on them," replies a third. "They wouldn't ever hurt you; you can always trust them."

Every time I ask this question the students hit the nail right on the head with their comments. "You guys got it right," I often say. "Clearly, a best friend is different from just a regular friend. A best friend is someone you've known much longer. He's someone that you have history with. You can look back over a pretty good chunk of time and see that a best friend wouldn't cheat you, wouldn't lie to you, and wouldn't do anything to deliberately try to hurt you. The length of time you have known your best friend allows you to evaluate that person much better. The more time goes by without a negative incident, the better able you are to get a sense of just how good a friend he is."

Then I'll ask, "How many of you have had a best friend who is no longer your best friend?" Only a couple of hands ever go up. To this day I get the same response: very few. Best friends are different from just ordinary friends. You love your best friends, you can trust them, they respect you and you respect them, and they usually stay in your life for a longer time than ordinary friends. Understanding what it takes to become—and stay—best friends with someone is the key that allows kids to understand when they have found love, respect, and trust in a romantic relationship.

When I conclude discussing the difference between friends and best friends, I segue back to my story about my wife. I tell the students that my wife became my best friend before we married and has been my best friend ever since. "I never have to worry that my wife will cheat on me or give me a sexually transmitted infection. I never have to fear that she would force me to have sex or hurt me if I chose not to. You see, my wife and I have true love, respect, and trust in our relationship. This kind of history is what you all need to have in a relationship with someone before you start to have sex."

How Can You Recognize Mutual Love, Respect, and Trust?

One of life's great challenges is to find a relationship with another person that offers these wonderful and endearing qualities. I suppose no one is perfect at knowing exactly when one has all this in a relationship; there are certainly plenty of people out there who must have thought they had it and got married, only to be divorced some time later. But I do know that we don't spend enough time as parents helping our children better understand love, respect, and trust. And this isn't the kind of thing we can expect our schools to help teach. Although there are probably no real "love, respect, and trust experts" out there, common sense informs us that if we allow our kids enough time to explore the characteristics of these qualities in meaningful and enlightened ways, they'll have a much better chance of recognizing the real deal when they find it. So please devote as much time as you can to talking with your kids about love, respect, and trust.

Below are some of the more important points that should help your kids identify when they have the "big three" ingredients in a relationship.

Imagine this conversation with your young son:

"Do you remember when our friend Ronni allowed her son Scott to go away for the weekend with his friends, and she said to him, 'I know you'll make the right decision and not drink alcohol while you are away. You're eighteen now and I trust you to make responsible decisions while on your own'? Well, Ronni had no idea whether or not Scott would drink alcohol, but she trusted him.

"You and I have spoken about how important trust is in a caring relationship with another person. When you trust someone, you never have to worry that she will make the wrong decision. A person that you trust is someone *you never worry about purposefully doing anything that could hurt or disappoint you.*

"Trust is also very important in a sexual relationship. I know we've talked about the type of person you would want to have a loving relationship with. Well, being able to trust the person would have to be a major ingredient in that relationship."

Time and Experience

The student who says she knows everything about her boyfriend after six months needs to be challenged. We all remember how much longer things seemed to take when we were kids. In a kid's mind, six months is a whole lot longer than it is in ours. We need to help our children understand that knowing someone for six months is better than knowing that person for three, but not as good as nine, or ten, or twelve months—or two or even three years, for that matter. We need to help our kids see how time and experience have a way of sorting things out for us, and when it comes to really getting to know someone, the more time the better.

We can do this by encouraging them to reflect on actual experiences that they have had where time played a role in helping them to better understand something, as I do when I discuss with students the difference between regular and best friends. Any examples like these will help our kids better understand how it takes time to determine if one loves another person, can trust that person, and has the respect of that person. So, for example, if you have your child reflect on what he knows today as opposed to the same time last year it will help to give him that perspective. Or if you discuss with your kid how he couldn't make a basket the first time he started playing basketball but two years later is on the all-star team, this should demonstrate how time and experience have allowed him to become a better player.

People who love, respect, and trust each other demonstrate this over time. These are not qualities that emerge after a short period of time; they evolve slowly and they cannot be rushed. In addition, people do not demonstrate these qualities for only a certain period of time; they consistently demonstrate them over and over again. This doesn't mean that they can't disagree or be angry or mad at each other. People who love, respect, and trust each other do have their moments that are rocky, but even during these times no one can deny that the "big three" still exist between them. However, if one cheats, lies, hurts, or denigrates his or her partner, then it is impossible to have real love, respect, and trust between them. No matter how much a person tries to show love, respect, and trust, there is no room for deliberately hurting one's partner—no room at all! You can't be super nice 95 percent of the time and purposefully hurt your partner the other 5 percent and expect to have true love, respect, and trust. It just doesn't work that way. Just as it is important to help your child understand when love, respect, and trust exist in a relationship, it is just as important to help your child develop an appreciation for when they don't.

Real Examples of Love, Respect, and Trust

This one is very simple: just take the time to highlight for your child examples of love, respect, and trust that occur in life. When your spouse or partner does something that exemplifies one of these traits, bring it to your child's attention. When you see these characteristics exhibited by your friends and neighbors, try to remember to tell your kids. Even when · you're watching television or a movie with your child and one of them is portrayed, bring it to your child's attention. These real-life examples need not be sexual; the "big three" are qualities you want your child to cherish in any loving and supportive relationship. Then, at a convenient time reflect back on one of these occurrences and point out how these qualities are especially important in a sexual relationship.

As your child gains reference points for the big three, she'll increase her ability to identify them when she personally experiences them. Any examples you can think of should be beneficial, but try to focus on those that highlight the big three in actual romantic relationships: someone going out of her way to do something for her partner out of love, someone sacrificing a personal desire out of respect for his partner's wishes, or someone allowing the partner to pursue something that requires the granting of considerable trust.

For example, if a friend of your husband stays overnight at a female colleague's apartment because he worked late and commuting home would take too long, you can discuss how your friend must really trust her husband not to "fool around." If someone you know agreed to put off having children for several years so that his partner could go to college and start a career, you can talk with your child about how much he must love his partner. If a friend totally disagrees with her partner's belief that their seventeen-year-old son should not be allowed to have friends over to the house while they are away for the night, but nevertheless doesn't overrule her partner, you can have a conversation about how that is an example of respect for her partner's position.

Use Authentic Teaching Strategies

I've spoken a lot already about authentic teaching; I cannot overstress that it is the most effective approach for teaching about sex and sexuality. Whatever we do as parents to help our children come to understand when one has love, respect, and trust, we must use authentic teaching strategies as part of our efforts. Let's look at some techniques that we could use:

Keep a Journal

Together with your child, keep a journal for a week. Both of you can enter different examples of how members of your family showed love, respect, and trust with each other. At the end of the week review the journal and explain why each of your entries is an example of the big three.

Tell a Story

Create a scenario that involves two sixteen-year-old kids who have been dating for two months. One evening after going to the movies they go over to a friend's house and they are hanging out in the backyard. After talking with their friends for a while, they wander over to the porch and start to kiss each other. After a minute or two, the boy puts his hand on his girlfriend's breast for the very first time. She is okay with it until he tries to slip his hand under her bra. She protests but the boy continues. She tries to push his hand away but he keeps forcibly touching her breast. She starts to cry but he keeps on doing it.

- Ask your child if it is possible that the boy respects the girl? Why or why not?
- Ask if the girl can trust the boy in the future? Why or why not?
- Should the girl continue to go out with the boy? Why or why not?

- What does this tell you about love, respect, and trust as they pertain to sex?

You should stress to your child why the answer to each of the first three questions is no. Because the boy did not stop and was actually forcing her to continue, he was absolutely wrong and she should not go out with him again. If he had stopped right away that would be another matter, but there must be no tolerance for one person forcing another person into sexual behavior. Explain that afterward the boy may be very remorseful and even ask for forgiveness, or he may even say that he only wanted to do it because he loves her, but that anyone who forces someone into any sort of sexual contact can't possibly have love or respect for that person. You can say that there are far too many people in relationships who experience abuse by their partners, and how this is a major problem in our society. You can also discuss with your child whether the girl should tell an adult what the boy tried to do.

Widen the Circle

The next time you are visiting relatives or good friends and your child is with you, tell them that you have been talking with your child about love, respect, and trust. Tell them that the two of you have been discussing how to tell when two people have these qualities in their relationship. Ask your relatives or friends to give an example or two of how they show love, respect, and trust in their relationship. Have your child give an example that she has noticed in their relationship.

Try a Role Reversal

Have your child pretend that he is your father (or your mother) and you are his child. Have him role-play with you what he would say about how to know when there is love, respect, and trust in a relationship with another. Be prepared to ask him questions that help clarify his statements.

Modeling

Along with authentic teaching, modeling for your children what a loving, respectful, and trustworthy relationship looks like can have an extremely powerful influence. We can do all the teaching that we possibly can about the big three, but, when we as parents can demonstrate on a day-to-day basis what these qualities look like, the impact on our children will be great. When love, respect, and trust are demonstrated by you and your partner it would be useful to periodically point it out to your children: "You know, what just happened between your father (or mother) and me is a perfect example of love (or respect or trust). I want you to remember what just took place because one day you are going to need to determine whether or not you are really in love with someone, and whether or not that person loves and respects you. This is not easy to do."

Even if you don't have a partner or spouse, there are still many opportunities where love, respect, and trust can be modeled. As an example, point out times when you or your children demonstrate these qualities for each other.

Love, Respect, and Trust: A Summation

I will focus a lot in this book on these three important qualities that are so necessary for any meaningful and lasting relationship. Of course, that is one of the major reasons why I want you to pay so much attention to them. But my interest in them really rests with my belief that they can insulate our children from some very nasty and horrible things. If we start early sending our message that love, respect, and trust should be established prior to being sexually active, and we repeat it often throughout their childhood, I am convinced that we can influence our children enough that they will remain abstinent until adulthood. So let's start thinking right now that we *can* do this for our kids.

Wouldn't it be wonderful if, because of the early intervention of all of the parents reading this book, we see a reduction in teen pregnancy, teen sexual abuse, and sexually transmitted infections? This *can* happen through the tremendous influence we gain with our children when we make the effort to become approachable. Strive to become the number one influence in your child's sexual life—because you do have the ability to bring about the sort of changes I am talking about here, more so than any sex education program.

If you are able to implement all that we have talked about up to this point, you can see how our kids are going to be in a very good place by the time they enter adolescence. This is because they will view us as approachable; they will have thought about sexual feelings and how to manage them; and they will have reflected on the relevance of love, respect, and trust in a relationship. As we continue with our efforts as our children travel through middle school and into high school, our influence should become noticeable in the sort of sexual behaviors our children will and will not engage in.

The importance of your efforts will become very clear in the next chapter, as we take an unflinching look at what's at stake. We will explore the importance of supporting and nurturing the positive and life-enhancing aspects of sex and sexuality, and the need to protect against the detrimental and dangerous consequences.

CHAPTER 4

What's at Stake: Understanding the Good and Bad Aspects of Sex

Perhaps the single most important message that your child needs to hear about sex is that it's like a coin, with two sides.

Without sex, none of us would be here today. Sex creates new life! Think about that. A microscopic sperm joins with an egg cell the size of a grain of sand and about nine months later a fully formed human being is born. Absolutely amazing! In my opinion, there is nothing more incredible than that fact.

But turn the coin over. Sex can kill you. What an interesting paradox: the same behavior that creates a life can also take a life!

Turn the coin back over. Sex can make two people who care deeply for one another feel even closer to each other. Physically rewarding intimacy with another person is something that so many of us want and seek, and when we experience it our lives can be thoroughly enhanced.

But turn the coin over again. The same behavior that has so enriched our lives can be catastrophic and horrible: witness teenage pregnancy, AIDS, sexual assault, sexual bullying, and the like.

After this chapter we're going to get pretty specific about what to say to your children, how to say it, when to say it, and the context in which to say it. We'll be talking sex probably like you've never done before. But first I want to talk to you more about this "sex is like a coin" paradox. I want you to fully appreciate the good and the bad aspects of sex because ultimately this is what we want our kids to be able to do. We want them to be able to make sense of a confusing sexual world and we want them to be able to distinguish between the good parts, the bad parts, and the ugly parts.

The Good

Well, thank goodness that there is a whole lot of good in sex and sexuality. And it's a message we do need to spread to our kids. But, as I said earlier, our discussions need to be balanced. I'm laughing inside as I write this because I'm thinking of the looks I've seen on the faces of the thousands of kids when I have told them that "sex can be good; it can be very good." It doesn't matter whether they're fourth graders or twelfth graders, most of them burst out laughing and look around at their classmates, not sure what to make of what I just said. Here's an adult who is telling them something that very few other adults, if any, have told them. But it is a message that they need to hear from an adult, in an honest, dignified, and mature context. Certainly most of them have gotten that message from plenty of sources of information *other* than a caring adult. Their sexualized wall is chock full of the "sex is great" message from music, DVDs, chat rooms, their peers, movies, and the like. But when I visit their classrooms, they are now going to hear that sex can be great from me. They are also going to hear many other important messages about sex from me (like being responsible, having empathy for others, being informed, and so on)—and without the BS from the media and all the other inaccurate sources of sexual information and influence. They also need to hear this from you!

As you know from the previous chapter, the three biggest sex words in this book are *love*, *respect*, and *trust*. Sex can be great when you have all three.

How Will You Know?

Admittedly, it's hard for any of us to truly know when we have love, respect, and trust in a relationship. Not surprisingly, too many high school kids have no clue about it either. "Oh, I'm in love, Dr. Fred. I've known him for six months and I know everything about him. He loves me; he'd never hurt me or leave me." Yeah, right, and I have some excellent swamp land to sell you! It sounds silly, but most of us have been there, haven't we? How many times did we think we were in love during high school?

So we need to spend a lot of time helping our child learn how to recognize the real thing. If we help kids understand love, respect, and trust, we'll reduce a lot of the *bad*. Even when kids know they should have these three things in a relationship—and *want* to have them— before they have sex, many are having sex because they *think* they've got those three qualities, when in reality they don't. If they understood this, I think many of them would rethink some of their sexual behavior. I could spend an entire year with these kids just exploring the signs and symptoms of having true love, respect, and trust in a relationship—it's such a complex issue and takes a long time to completely understand.

You will want to instill in your children that they are sexual human beings and will be so until the day they die—that they will experience a variety of sexual emotions as they grow and develop, and that those emotions are normal and part of being human. I always tell kids and parents that the single most significant change of puberty has nothing to do with biological changes; it is the development of sexual feelings. Our sexual feelings represent a major aspect of who we are, and we must help our kids understand how to manage and negotiate them, and teach them to appreciate the positive value they can add to one's life.

So now I want you to think of your kid at age fifteen, sixteen, and seventeen. Will you be comfortable with her having sexual intercourse at one of these ages? Let us assume that she is smart and aware, and appears to pretty much understand how to handle herself in a romantic relationship. Let's also say that she has known her partner for several years and is certain there is love, respect, and trust between them. Will you be comfortable knowing that she is having sex as a minor? If so, please be very certain that you read this entire book and follow my advice on how to prepare your child to protect herself from sexual harm. You need to remember that adults sure make enough mistakes when it comes to their sexual relationships, and because of their age and immaturity teens are even more likely to make mistakes. In light of this, are you going to be okay with your sixteen-year-old doing it? How about your seventeen-year-old? I'm not saying that there could never be circumstances in which you'd be comfortable knowing your teenager is sexually intimate. I'm just saying you should think long and hard before you are okay with the prospect of your teen being sexually active.

You also want your children to appreciate the sobering magnitude of the creation of new life as well as just how miraculous it is. This is another major aspect of real life that most schools spend virtually no time on. How do we as a society allow our public schools to not spend any significant time helping our children learn to appreciate the complex set of responsibilities that are necessary in order to have a baby? That's not to say that there aren't some noteworthy parenting education programs in public schools. There are. I've seen classes dedicated to parenting, kids carrying "baby eggs" or sacks of flour around with the instructions to treat them like actual babies so they get a feel for what it might be like to have a real baby, and some students learn about real babies and their parents who visit their classrooms so they better understand child development and parent-child relationships. But believe me, these programs are rare and usually relegated to our high schools. I would say that the overwhelming majority of students never experience any parenting education in their entire school career, and those who do have more fingers on their hands than hours spent learning about the subject. I believe this to be the case even in those school districts that have state regulations requiring parent education for students.

Like I said previously, on paper an educational system can indicate that it provides something to students but in actuality do so in a very limited fashion. One of the most important things that most humans will do in life is try to be a good parent, and our schools spend virtually zero time on anything remotely resembling parenting education. So it is up to us parents to help our children to develop the skills that are needed to postpone pregnancy until adulthood, put the miracle of life into a context that they can understand, and gain some semblance of what is needed for parenthood.

The Bad

Unfortunately, there are far too many bad aspects of sex. I'll lay out for you the problematic and troubling side of sexual behavior that you will want to pay close attention to.

The Sexual Bully

In my opinion, the scariest trend in child sexual behavior in recent years is sexual bullying: children harassing, intimidating, even assaulting others by using some form of sexual behavior or by provoking another child to use some form of unwanted sexual behavior.

"We are raising a generation of sexualized bullies," I tell a large group of elementary school parents at one of the public schools that I work with. "As we sexualize all children through the vast array of sources of sexual information and influences, we are also sexualizing those children who are becoming bullies. And these developing bullies are learning that using sexual behavior to bully other children is as effective, if not more so, than using traditional methods of bullying. I get numerous calls from elementary school principals, counselors, and other school staff about young children who are using sexual behavior to harass, intimidate, and strike fear in other children. We almost never saw these behaviors among such young children in previous decades. But now we are seeing them on a regular basis. So beware the sexual bully."

The parents stare back at me in amazement. Most of them are shocked to hear me say this. Some, however, nod their heads in agreement and acknowledge that their own child or a friend's child has been bullied in such a way. Lately, more and more parents know what I am talking about. I get far too many calls about children who touch the genitals of other children without consent, and force them to touch their genitals in return. There are children who force other children to pull their pants down, children who intimidate other children by rubbing their genitals against them or by lying on top of them. There are children who will forcefully kiss another child's genitals or force them to kiss their own.

Both the perpetrators and the victims can be as young as five, six, or seven years of age. Again, we are now seeing these behaviors far too frequently. When a parent comes forward in one of my presentations and acknowledges that her child has been sexually touched in an intrusive or hurtful manner by another child, it takes a whole lot of courage. I can only imagine how many more remain silent. This is what happens when children have multiple exposures to sexualized messages that are confusing and incomprehensible to them. The sexual bully has been created as a result and will remain as long as we live in a hypersexualized society.

Online Harassment

I have dealt far too often with students who have been humiliated and devastated as a result of "sexting" and harassment while online. Some of these kids are as young as ten and eleven, and countless more are of middle school age. Tragically, we have even seen children commit suicide as a result of this type of harassment. This tells us that as parents we need to begin our discussions of sexting and online dangers with our kids while they are still in elementary school.

Targeting Specific Sexualities

Discrimination against, and persecution of, gay, lesbian, bisexual, and transgender youth by other youth is a very significant problem in our society. Irrespective of what one believes about homosexuality or differing sexualities, there is no room for discrimination or persecution. Unfortunately, there are people who are bullied, harmed, and even killed because their sexuality is perceived as something other than heterosexual. The message our kids need to hear from all of us is that we must never treat those who seem to be different with any less respect than the way we expect to be treated.

Understanding the Sexual Bully

One truly frightening potential of hypersexualizing children is an increase in numbers of adolescent and adult sexual offenders. We have known for a long time that the origins of hurtful sexual behavior, in fact the origins of any violent behavior, occur very early in life. Most adult sexual offenders began to develop their perpetrator behavior as young children, and retrospective studies reveal that a majority of adult sexual offenders committed their first offenses as adolescents.[1] This raises the question of what will happen if we continue to see an increasing number of sexual bullies who are children. Will we see more sexual offenders down the road?

I think we know the answer to this question. Sadly, I have already seen far too many cases of sexualized bullying that have occurred in schools.[2] My most recent case of sexualized bullying was a six-year-old girl who was caught—several times—touching the penises of boys her age on the bus on the way to school. One day, a boy in her grade told his teacher that the girl was bothering him. When asked what she was doing he would only say, "She just keeps bothering me." Eventually, his teacher drew out of him that the girl had "touched his privates." And the girl freely admitted to asking the boy if she could touch him. In fact, she calmly and matter-of-factly described what she had done. When asked why she'd done it, she just replied, "I don't know." Her mother was informed and expressed concern but said she couldn't imagine why her daughter would have done such a thing.

The girl was caught a second time and said, "It was an accident." But when the behavior occurred a third time, the school asked the mother to have her daughter seen by a mental health practitioner. Unfortunately the mother did not follow through and shortly thereafter another boy came forward. Only this time, the girl had licked his penis. The boy said she'd been touching it and then had asked him if she could lick it "like a lollipop." He told the teacher he'd initially refused, but that she had continued to ask until he eventually relented.

It was at this point that the situation was brought to my attention, and I had the case referred to the child protection agency. An investigation found that the girl, who lives in a city-funded temporary shelter, had witnessed numerous sexual encounters between her mother and the mother's boyfriend. I am happy to say that the little girl is now receiving very good mental health care and I am hopeful that this intervention will halt any further development of her sexualized bullying behavior. She does, however, still require an adult escort on the school bus to monitor her behavior.

Unfortunately, I have far too many stories like this to share. Some involve group sexual activities, invariably organized by one child who is the bully. He or she develops or determines what sexual activities the group will engage in: usually touching behaviors that involve the genitals. At times, the behavior may escalate to include humping or oral-genital contact. Other students are recruited through coercion or fear in order to ensure the activities are carried out. The bully will punish any member of the group who tries to disrupt the activities. Sometimes the sexual bully actually befriends the other children, and will only use intrusive tactics when he or she has to.

I have also handled many cases that involve only one-child-at-a-time bullying. The sexual bully who orchestrates group sex needs to keep multiple children involved, which requires a front of friendly seduction for recruiting. The one-on-one sexual bully doesn't have to manage multiple players to make things happen, so he or she can afford to use a more coercive and fear-inducing tactic. If it doesn't work, the bully can easily go on to another child. While the group-oriented sexual bully tends to make a game out of his or her bullying, the one-on-one sexual bully typically gets straight to the bullying. This usually includes intrusive, dominating, and offensive sexual touching, which may or may not lead to more adult-like sexual behavior.

As parents, we should always be ready and able to evaluate our children's sexual behaviors; particularly those that involve another child. Are you capable of doing that? For example, the "I'll show you mine if you show me yours" game has been around forever. So when you catch your seven-year-old child on a playdate where he and his playmate have their pants down, giggling and embarrassed, it is probably a normal expression of sexual curiosity. When children display a genuine sense of sexual curiosity, they do it with a great deal of natural wonder, which is often accompanied by embarrassment.

When the behavior becomes problematic, you can usually tell by paying attention to the context in which it occurs. That means that if a sexual behavior appears to cause fear, concern, anxiety, or stress, then it's probably unwanted and you need to be on guard. Naturally occurring sexual curiosity between children does not produce these effects.

If you notice that your child displays any of the following, he or she may be a victim of sexual bullying:

- Fear of being left alone with a particular child
- Nightmares or sleep problems with no explanation
- In an older child, regression to behavior such as thumb-sucking or bed-wetting
- Resistance to routine bath time activities, using the toilet, or removing clothes in otherwise appropriate situations

If your child or another child you know engages in the following it could be indicative of sexual bullying:

- Responding sexually to ordinary gestures of friendliness or affection
- Insisting on physical contact with a child even when that child resists

- Turning to younger or less-powerful children rather than peers to explore natural sexual curiosity
- Taking younger children to "secret" places to play "special" undressing or touching games
- Displaying interest in sexual matters beyond what you would expect for the child's age, or engaging in sexual behavior on an excessive or compulsive basis

In addition, there are some sexual behaviors that in and of themselves cause concern. Here are some warning signs and sexual behaviors that call for your intervention:

- Sexual behavior engaged in excessively, or to the exclusion of other activities
- Genital touching of another child where there is actual manipulation or massaging of the genitals (beyond the single tentative touch of curiosity)
- Sexual behavior involving age disparity or difference in power between the children
- Any attempt to engage in sexual intercourse or simulate sexual intercourse
- Any attempt to engage in oral sex
- Any attempt to insert objects into the rectum or vagina

So what do you do if you happen to observe any of these behaviors? The last group listed requires immediate action. These are behaviors that by themselves should cause us concern and require intervention by a qualified mental health provider. For those behaviors that could indicate that the child is a victim of sexual bullying, keep in mind that any of these occurrences, on its own, doesn't automatically mean something is happening to your child. But an overall pattern of behavior involving more than one of these issues is something to address with your child's doctor or a mental health professional.

When talking to your child about what's going on, stress that it is not his or her fault, and acknowledge your child's courage in being willing to talk about it. Reinforce that you are there to love and protect your child. Above all, stay calm and keep your own emotions in check. For those behaviors that might indicate sexual bullying, you will want to take action. If your own child is bullying, it means calling a mental health professional; if it is another child, it means calling their parents and, if these behaviors are occurring at school, the school authorities. Keep in mind that anytime a child is engaging in sexual bullying there is the possibility that the behavior is against the law. The idea that legal authorities could be called with regard to a child's behavior can be difficult to come to terms with. But remember that this is sometimes the only way to get help for the parties involved—help that can heal a victim and hopefully lead to treatment and support for the perpetrator so he or she will stop the behavior.

If we are vigilant we can really make a difference in reducing the incidence of child sexual bullying and the display of problematic sexual behavior. Clearly, we must first know which sexual behaviors may be problematic—which is why I listed the warning signs on pages 68–69. When we can recognize sexual behaviors that stray from what we would normally see in children, we stand a better chance of intercepting the development of problematic sexual behavior. And always keep in mind the following: fear, coercion, force, stress, or anxiety; one child older or more powerful than another; and sexual behaviors that seem excessive or are not stopped when boundaries are set. These are all warning signs. And, of course, any sexual behavior that reflects that of adults—real or simulated intercourse, oral sex, or insertion of objects into the rectum or vagina—is problematic.

MONKEY SEE, MONKEY DO

The sexual bully is just one manifestation of a general problem: kids are simply acting out what they are exposed to. It makes sense that the more times a child is confronted with confusing sexualized messages, the likelier it becomes that he will experience more and more difficulty managing those messages. Consequently, the more explicit the sexual messages are and the more frequently they are consumed by the child, the more likely it is that the child will manifest some problem as a result of all the exposure. One of the most common problems arises when the child acts out the sexual behaviors he has been exposed to.

Consequently, some children will become sexual bullies. Others will try to engage other children in sexual behaviors but without the level of coercion we see with the sexual bully. Still others simply become confused by what they see and hear. No doubt virtually all these children will require some sort of adult intervention to help them make sense of what they have been exposed to. Many of them will require a more intensive, therapeutic intervention to help them resolve their confusion, stop their sexualized behavior, and return to a healthier place.

Teen Sexual Intercourse, Pregnancy, and STDs

While I believe that our message about sex to our kids has got to be balanced, that is, sex positive and sex negative, we have to be clear with our kids that we hope they remain abstinent until adulthood. That doesn't mean that a little "foolin' around" is necessarily bad. When I say this I do so with the understanding that it is normal during adolescence to want to express physical affection, and when teens do so we shouldn't overreact by viewing it as problematic. I'll clarify this in chapter 9 by discussing how parents can determine when physical affection among teens becomes too risky. For now, let me just say that we need to start early with our message about two major principles: not having any type of sexual intercourse until adulthood, and then only in a context of true respect, trust, and love in his or her relationship. So remember these words: *love*, *respect*, and *trust*, for they are by far the most important sex words in any book on sex.

I get many calls from school counselors who ask my advice on eleven-, twelve-, and thirteen-year-old kids who are engaging in sexual intercourse. When I get one of these calls, two sides of myself become instantly concerned. One, obviously, is the professional sex educator in me. I immediately begin to work with the counselor to develop a plan of intervention. Our goals are (1) to help this young person develop the capacity to make better decisions about sexual behavior, and (2) to try to determine the reasons why a decision to have sex was made. Every case is unique, yet we do see patterns. Some of the contributing factors that lead to early sexual intercourse are chaotic family life; abuse; alcohol; destructive peer group and peer pressure; mental illness like depression, conduct disorder, and oppositional defiance disorder; poor self-esteem and self-concept; and just poor decision making.

The father in me is the other part of myself that jumps to attention. I immediately think of my own kid and what I would need to do as a parent to ensure that this never happens to him. The ultimate reality for a parent is that you can't completely control what behavior your child will engage in. But when I receive a call from a counselor who is concerned about a child engaging in sexual intercourse, I also think of all the things I need to do as a parent to minimize the chances that my child would engage in risky and destructive behavior. So very often, I see actions that parents have taken or not taken that have contributed to their child's early sexual activity, and when I am looking at one of these cases, I too must come to terms with my own failings as a parent.

What Part Do I Play?

My point is that every one of us must take full responsibility for being a parent. Irrespective of our own personal life dilemmas, we need to constantly ask ourselves, *What am I not doing for my kids that I should be doing? How can I be better at serving my children?* Our kids didn't choose us as parents. But we are the parents they got. All parents, regardless of socioeconomic, cultural, and racial backgrounds, fall somewhere on a spectrum from effective to ineffective. And you need to ask yourself, *Where do I fall?*

Ironically, our own children need to be asking themselves similar questions as they grow and develop. *How do I as a girl or boy manage my life so that I grow up to be a healthy, happy, capable adult?* And specifically with respect to sexual behavior, *How do I ensure that I get to enjoy the good, life-enhancing, satisfying aspects of sex and sexuality, and avoid the destructive, horrible, and even deadly aspects?* This brings us back to the "sex is like a coin" analogy I spoke about previously. As parents we need to ask, at every stage of our child's development, *What is it that I need to instill in my child about the good and bad aspects of sex and sexuality?*

Laying the Foundation: Early Lessons

Let's start with helping them avoid the negative consequences; here are a few examples:

- You explain and reinforce to your four- and five-year-olds that no one is allowed to touch their private parts and they are not allowed to touch the private parts of others. Again, you clearly explain the exceptions—Mom or Dad teaching them how to wash their private parts, or a doctor examining their private parts to make sure they stay healthy—but otherwise it's hands off.

- When your eight-year-old is watching a news story about HIV infection, you interject with a broader discussion of how there are many other types of infections one can spread through sexual intercourse.

- When your ten-year-old hears that the thirteen-year-old in the apartment down the hall is pregnant, you seize the opportunity to discuss strategies to avoid an unwanted pregnancy.

When I talk to ten-year-olds, I work with them to explore why far too many kids in this country become pregnant every year and how there can be epidemic levels of sexually transmitted infections among teenagers. No matter where I encounter fifth graders, very few have any sort of deep awareness of the personal and social costs of teenage pregnancy, and there are even fewer who appreciate the costs of sexually transmitted infections; HIV and AIDS don't cause nearly the level of concern they did just ten years ago. Most kids of this age know very little about all that can happen to them if they become sexually active. When I tell parents that the incidence of teen sexual activity goes from about 8 to 10 percent for seventh graders to almost 32 percent for ninth graders, their eyes open pretty wide.[3] If you have a kid in elementary school and you wait until middle school to have in-depth discussions about intercourse, it may be too late. It takes a good deal of time to learn how to drive a car, but it takes much longer to become a very good driver. How long do you think it takes a teenager to learn how to manage and control their sexual emotions and feelings?

Oral Sex Is Sex

Our discussion of sexual intercourse must include oral sex and anal sex. When I talk to both students and parents I am very emphatic about this. If you're going to put your mouth on a vulva or on a penis, you had darn well better come to terms with the fact that you are having sex. The same goes for anal sex. We do believe that oral sex is about as widespread as vaginal sex among teens ages fifteen to seventeen, and the incidence of anal sex for this age group is between 6 and 7 percent.[4] It's worth noting that there is great difficulty in obtaining various data about the sexual behaviors of minors. There are legal and ethical dilemmas involved with trying to survey minors about the sort of sexual behaviors they engage in. Countless kids have told me that oral sex is not sex. There is a pervasive belief that they are still virgins if they have oral sex, and far too many still believe that one cannot contract HIV orally. "What, are you kidding me?" I say to them. "Of course it's sex. And about that idea of still being a virgin? Forget it—if you put your mouth on it, or if your girlfriend or boyfriend puts her or his mouth on your genitals, you can throw the virgin idea out the window. You all need to realize that whether it's vaginal sex or oral sex, it's all sex."

The Ugly

You'll notice that some of the things I categorize as the *ugly* could also be categorized as the *bad*. That is, all of the ugly is bad, but may not necessarily be as bad as what I discussed in that section. I'll cover this issue in more detail later in the book, but when I say *ugly*, I'm talking about things like the following:

- Girls who dress in a sexy way—or at least want to—at a very young age. Too many ten-, eleven-, and twelve-year-old girls are trying to appear far older than they are
- Sexual harassment through suggestive comments, stares, and gestures—mainly boy to girl, but also girl to boy, girl to girl, and boy to boy
- "Sexting" and social media networking

- Music and DVDs that are demeaning to women (especially) and to men

And, of course:

- Boys who let their pants hang low and look like slobs

These are some of the *ugly* aspects of sex that I'll address later in the book.

It's time now to talk about an issue that, while it may seem frivolous to some, can make all the difference in raising kids who understand and appreciate their bodies—and who will defend them from harm. I'm talking about all the "secret" body parts and the silly or ugly slang terms we use for these parts and their functions. I'll explain why our kids can and should use the real words, from the start.

CHAPTER 5

It's a Penis, Not a Doohickey

I didn't know I had a penis until I was ten. For many years I honestly thought my penis was called a *doohickey* because that was what my father called it. Sometimes he would mix it up and call it a *pee-pee*, and I suppose when he was feeling really frisky he'd call it a *dick*. But whatever my father said it was called, I believed him. And I bet that's the way it was for most of the men reading this book. Were you told it was called a *penis*? Probably not.

I clearly remember, when I was about eight, my dad telling me, "Hey, got to protect your doohickey, Fred," before taking me out to the ball field and hitting endless baseballs to me at first base. "You never know when you might get one in your doohickey," he'd always remind me. "You got to make sure you wear your protective cup every time you go out and play." I imagine he wanted me to protect my testicles more than he did my penis, but strangely enough he never said the word *testicles* or, for that matter, *balls*. So I learned early in life I had a *doohickey*, but I remained *ball*-less for a number of years thereafter. Go figure.

Why Not Use Slang?

You may be thinking, *Sure, I do this—but* all *parents do this*. We allow our kids to learn all these alternative names for their private parts except the ones that they should be learning. We have our reasons (embarrassment over the real terms, mostly), but the bigger question is what harm, if any, do we do when we use slang words for our sexual and reproductive body parts? I'm guessing most of you would reply, *Very little harm.* "So you call the testicles *balls*, the vagina a *cunt*, the penis a *prick*, and the breasts *tits*. What's the big deal?" you may ask. You may have a similar reaction to terms for various sexual behaviors. So if sexual intercourse becomes *fucking*, and oral sex becomes *giving head*, and anal sex becomes *bone smuggling*, and masturbation becomes *awaken the bacon*, you may think that's no big deal either. "They're only words," you may say. But it's very important for parents to think about how "only words" play out over time with the thinking of young kids.

Let's go back to our children's sexualized wall of messages for a moment. When kids learn early on that there are dozens of slang names for their sexual and reproductive body parts, and we allow those words to become part of their lexicon without insisting that they learn to use the more socially accepted terms, we send them the message that there is something shameful about those body parts. That for whatever reason they can't be spoken about unless we substitute some other name. This creates several serious problems. One concerns children who have been sexually abused. We know there are some children who will not report their abuse because they have learned that they shouldn't say those words or have learned to associate a sense of shame with anything having to do with their private parts. Think about that for a moment: because we often fail to teach our kids the proper names for their genitalia, a number of sexually abused children remain silent.

Down and Dirty

Another problem with using sexual slang is that children fail to develop a sense of dignity around sexual matters. This means that things pertaining to sex remain "dirty" and are something that we just shouldn't talk about. As a result, many children and young people are uncomfortable with communicating honestly and openly about sex and sexuality. And this discomfort perpetuates poor communication about sex between parents and their children. It even contributes to a lack of communication between teenagers and young adults who get involved in sexual relationships, which in turn can contribute to irresponsible sexual decision making. But perhaps the most pervasive consequence of using slang terminology is its effect, over time, of stripping away the lovemaking aspect of sexual intercourse and other sexually intimate acts. At times it seems as though members of our society don't make love anymore—we simply fuck each other. And when this happens, we no longer require the love, trust, and respect that come with and from lovemaking.

In addition, kids who grow up with the slang also tend to objectify another person's sexual body parts, making a person's sexual parts the focus of their interest. When you do that, it's easy to lose sight of the total person, to make their genitals the object of conquest. Statements like "I'm gonna hit that pussy," "Let's tap that ass," and "I'm gonna ride that locker room terror" reduce sexual intimacy to the use of power and control of another person's body.

Ignorance Is Not Bliss

I can go into any third- or fourth-grade class today and I'll guarantee you that 75 percent won't have a clue what testicles are. But if I use the word *balls* they will all know. Learning the slang, however, is only part of the problem. There are many sexual parts of the body that many kids don't even know exist. I know of very few fifth graders who know what a urethra is, and I bet that most fifth-grade boys think a woman urinates from her vagina. Heck, most eighth-grade boys probably think that too. I was in a fifth-grade class just recently and asked the students what part of a female's body produces egg cells. "The stomach," "the part that holds a baby," they answered. Not one knew it was the ovaries. And I have found that it really doesn't matter which community I visit or the particular set of demographics that exist there. Kids are pretty much ignorant of sexual anatomy irrespective of their socioeconomic status, race, culture, and other factors. In fact, if I asked you to draw the sexual and reproductive parts of a male and female, and label each part, I'd wager that you would fail the test. So where does that leave our kids?

So simply teaching our children to use the actual names for their sexual and reproductive body parts, as well as the actual names for different sexual acts, will go a long way toward enabling them to communicate effectively about sex and sexuality. By discouraging their use of slang terminology, we increase their chances of gaining a more healthy and life-enhancing view of sex and sexuality. Of course, your child will still learn the slang terminology and be exposed to the debasement that comes from using and hearing it; many of his peers will use it, and your child will hear it many times through various media outlets. This is inescapable. But by reinforcing the use of proper language and discouraging its misuse, you can minimize your child's chances of incorporating slang terminology into his or her lexicon, and you'll help your child develop a sense of dignity around sex and sexuality.

If you don't want your young kid using the slang, you need to do two important things at the appropriate ages: (1) teach your child the correct terms that rightfully belong in their sexual and anatomical vocabulary, and (2) teach your child the sexual slang words you *don't* want them saying. That's right—as you will see shortly, you will have to have some discussion about the words you don't want your child to use.

Safety First: Private Parts for Little Ones

All three-year-olds should know the words for their genitals and private parts of their body. No ifs, ands, or buts! (No pun intended.) So let's see: *penis, testicles, breasts, vulva, clitoris,* and *vagina*. For kids three and four years old, these are the basics; the rest can come later. Just as you would teach your child about any of his other body parts, so will you teach him about his private parts and genitals. Make your discussions brief, as young children's attention span is limited, and don't make it seem like it's a big deal to be learning about them. When you're dressing her or bathing him, you can go through a list of different body parts including their private parts: "You know, your body is very special and there are a lot of different parts to it. You have your arms, legs, neck, and head; and you have a penis, testicles, and buttocks." You can point to each part and then say, "Some parts of our bodies are private and some of them are public." You can have a similar discussion with your daughter: "These folds between your legs are your vulva, the opening between them is your vagina, and just above your vagina is a little button-size body part called the clitoris. These are your buttocks, behind you, and these are your nipples up here on your chest."

Connecting private parts with private places is a very important concept to teach your children: "Your vagina, clitoris, breasts, and buttocks are the parts of your body that can only be shown in private places like your bedroom and the bathroom. When you go outside you always cover your private parts."

This can be confusing, as we have a tendency to let our little ones run around naked every once in a while at the beach, outside in the yard, and various other places. But in the United States kids need to learn a sense of sexual modesty as they get older. For most kids, and from a developmental standpoint, this usually happens by the age of eight. For little girls, their breasts are not as private as they will be when they begin to grow and develop. Feel free to say to your little five- or six-year-old girl, "Your breasts are private now. No one should touch them but it's okay sometimes for little girls to not cover their breasts all the time. When your breasts start to grow when you get older, you will have to cover them. I know that may be a little hard to understand, but that is just the way it is."

You also want to address the much more important issue of others touching a child's private parts. Just as we establish rules for behavior with our children around the house, in public, or at school, we need to establish rules concerning private parts: "A rule that you need to live by is no one is allowed to touch your private parts except Mommy or Daddy, and we will only do so when we wash you, or if we have to put medicine on your private parts, for example. Or sometimes your doctor has to look at and touch your private parts to make sure that you are healthy or if you are hurting there. But those are the only exceptions." Just as important is the concept that they are not allowed to touch the genitals or private parts of another person: "Just like the rule that no one should touch your private parts, we have another rule that says you shouldn't touch anyone else's—and there are no exceptions."

Begin Early and Keep Building

This is a lot of important information, and you will disseminate it according to how much your little one can absorb. But you do need to start this discussion by age three—and you need to keep repeating it. You will also *scaffold* your talks—that is, build on and expand the information you offer. As your child learns each concept and gets to understand each topic you broach, you can add on more information and guidance, just as a builder raises the scaffolding as he builds each story of a building. So, for example, when your son is three you tell him the name of his testicles; when he is five, you briefly discuss the purpose of his testicles—that is, they will make sperm cells, and when a sperm cell joins with an egg cell a new life is created. Somewhere in the age span of five to eight you describe how that occurs through sexual intercourse. We will discuss this in far greater detail shortly.

You do want your son to learn about the private body parts of a girl, and you want your daughter to learn about the private body parts of a boy. It has to work both ways; girls should learn what the boys learn and boys should learn what the girls learn. Not only are children naturally curious about the differences between girls and boys at this age—and in short order they will need to understand the very basic process of reproduction and how babies are made—but they also need to understand that both genders have private parts: "Boys don't have a vagina, they have a penis. The penis looks a little like a soft noodle, and, when a boy urinates, urine comes out of the tip of his penis." "Girls don't have a penis; they have a vagina, which is an opening between their legs. They don't urinate from their vagina like a boy does from his penis. There is a tiny opening right near their vagina where the urine comes out." If you wish, feel free to go to the library for an age-appropriate children's book that shows some nicely done drawings of different body parts.

Find Your Teaching Style

I believe it is important to qualify with your child that these discussions are meant to be discussed privately between the two of you, and that it's not okay to talk about this stuff with other people. You know how little kids can be, blithely sharing everything that you've talked about with other people. So set some boundaries for your talks with your child.

You also need to determine just how often you want to have these discussions with your child and how much you'll say when you do. Use any teachable moments that you can. If, for example, you and your child are watching television and you see a scene that depicts a young child needing to go to her parents for help, you can say something like, "Remember, just like that girl on TV, you should always tell Mommy or Daddy if someone tries to harm you. Like if someone tries to touch your private parts."

Or when you are bathing your son, you can say, "Remember, aside from Mommy or Daddy helping you wash your private parts or having the doctor examine your private parts, no one is allowed to touch them."

This is one issue that you will need to discuss more than most. Young kids need to hear the rules about the touching of private parts a number of times. They need to understand what they should do if someone tries to touch them or when someone else tries to get them to touch, and they need to know that they should always tell you or another trusted adult when someone tries to do this to them. You don't want to scare them, so don't overstate your message, but do plan to discuss this to some degree throughout their childhood and teenage years.

Being Naked Around Your Little One

Walking around naked in front of your little one is something that most all of us have done. Bathing with them, dressing with them, or walking around your house in front of them in the buff is no big deal. But you should talk with them at some point to clarify the rules: because this is Mommy and Daddy, it is okay to be naked, but we don't walk around nude in public or in front of other people. Don't worry that you might be scaring them from one day ever disrobing in front of others, say, when in a locker room. They will no doubt come to learn the distinction in due time—that is, kids will be exposed to numerous situations in life that will help them see that there are gradations of the concepts of "private" and "public." For example, one can be very private in the privacy of one's bathroom but cannot always be in the privacy of a public bathroom. Nevertheless, you will inevitably end your moments of nudity with your kids at some point. Either your kids will stop wanting to disrobe in front of you anymore, which will likely occur around eight years of age or so, or you yourself will become uncomfortable being naked in front of them.

Sometimes little ones can be quite obnoxious with their behavior when we are nude around them. Every now and again we come across one who simply loves bugging the crap out of us—you know, the little son or daughter who just delights in poking us in our buttocks, penis, or breasts. It may happen once, twice, or three times, but at some point it becomes really annoying. If you have a child who is a poker or a grabber, my suggestion is to get a handle on his behavior right away and make it stop, or things could get a little out of hand. There's nothing cute about a child grabbing or poking your (or anyone else's) private parts. When it happens even once, I would intervene. You want to label the behavior, tell your child how the behavior makes you feel, and set limits: "When you poke Mommy in the breast like that it hurts, and I don't want you to do that again." Or, "When you grab Daddy's penis it can hurt. There is nothing funny about doing that; you must not do that anymore." Make sure you acknowledge any positive behavior moving forward, as you want to reward behavior that is acceptable. If your child stops engaging in the behavior for a day or so, you want to say something like, "You haven't poked Mommy in the buttocks today. I am proud of your behavior." Always make sure you reward "good" behavior.

What if My Little One Asks Me . . .

So when you teach your three- or four-year-old the words *testicles*, *vagina*, *penis*, and *breasts*, what do you say if she asks, *What do these parts do?* or, *Why do we have them?* It is unlikely that your child will ask these questions at this age, but so what if she does ask? It's not a big deal; you just calmly answer the questions. *Some of the answers are gonna get us into a sex talk, and my kid is just too young for that*, you may be thinking. Keep in mind that these little ones really couldn't care less about sex, so giving them a little insight into it is not going to cause any harm. What it will do is open the door to your *becoming an approachable parent for your child*. Your child will learn early on that she can come to you for any guidance on the subject of sex. After all, that is your goal.

But let's assume for a moment that your kid does ask how all this happens. What's a natural response? If your child asks why boys have testicles, your response could be, "They produce sperm cells." My guess is your child will just say, "Oh," and move on. If, however, he asks what sperm cells are for, you can respond, "They help to make a baby." Should he ask how that happens, you can say, "A sperm cell from the father joins with an egg cell from the mother and that makes a baby." What if the child asks how the sperm meets the egg? You can say, "The father puts his penis into the mother's vagina and the sperm cells come out of the father's penis. There is an egg cell in the mother's body and the sperm joins with it to make a baby."

I hope you haven't just fainted. I know, it seems hard to have a frank discussion like this with your young child. But honestly, if your conversation with your three- or four-year-old gets this far, it is likely your kid will be fast asleep out of sheer boredom. And if for some reason he is not asleep, I am sure he will view the whole process as disgusting and will not want to hear any more about it. Irrespective of which response your child makes, you will want to close your conversation with something along the following lines: "Now, remember, this is private talk between Mommy (or Daddy) and you. We do not talk about private parts with other people. But I want you to know that if you have more questions about this you can always come to Mommy (or Daddy) and ask. You know we love you very much and you can ask us anything."

For questions about the vagina or penis and what its function is, you can adapt the responses I gave above. I suppose you could opt for a "safer" response by saying, "The penis is the part of a man's body that allows urine to come out." Or, "The vagina is the opening between a woman's legs that allows a baby to come out when it is ready to be born." Just remember that eventually (and certainly by age eight) you will need to discuss these body parts in relation to intercourse and reproduction. If your child asks about women's breasts and why they are bigger than a man's you can say, "A woman's breasts are bigger than a man's because in order to breast-feed the baby the mother's breasts need to be big enough so the baby can drink milk from them. Mommies have milk in their breasts after they give birth and many of them breast-feed their baby. So that is why their breasts need to be bigger." Again, the odds are very much in your favor that your child will not ask any further questions. But you do need to remember the basic rule: we never ignore one of our child's questions. So we all need to be ready with answers.

Beyond the Basics with Your Slightly Older Little Ones

It's always interesting to watch five- and six-year-olds hear me discuss with them the names for their private parts. I always make sure to do this with their teacher by my side so as to make them feel as safe and comfortable as possible. When you say the words *penis, vagina, clitoris, testicles, ovaries,* and *breasts* in front of a class of twenty-five first or second graders, you are bound to get a bunch of reactions. Invariably, you will always have some children whose eyes become as wide as humanly possible, some with big smiles across their faces, a few whose mouths fall open with the most incredulous looks, and those who will actually fall back on the floor while sitting in their circle on the rug. And believe it or not there are always a few students who will actually handle my talk with more maturity than their parents would.

My advice for your discussion of private parts with a five- or six-year-old is similar to that for the three- or four-year-old. You will want to periodically review the different names for the genitals and private parts of a woman and a man, and you will also want to review your safety rules having to do with avoiding abuse. But with a five- or six-year-old, I recommend that you also discuss some of the functions of the various body parts, if you haven't already. For example, I would say to this group, "The body is made up of many, many cells. Cells are very tiny but when many of them are put together they actually form different parts of a body. This is what happens when a baby is growing inside the uterus of her mother. There are cells that make the arms and legs, cells that make the chest, cells that make the bones, cells that make the heart and lungs, and cells that make up the entire body. Both girls and boys have the same type of cells except for one particular type of cell. There is one type of cell that a man has that a woman doesn't have, and one type of cell that a woman has that a man doesn't have. The man has sperm cells and the woman has egg cells. And they're all very, very small. The testicles make sperm cells. Just as a man has two testicles, a woman has two ovaries that make the eggs. The ovaries are inside a woman's body. When a sperm cell from the father joins together with an egg cell from the mother, it makes a baby." No doubt some of these five- and six-year-olds, like their younger counterparts, will be totally bored at this point. Few, if any, will ask how the sperm cell gets together with the egg cell, but if they do, you will answer it the same way we did with the three- and four-year-olds.

You'll also want to explain what a uterus is. No, the baby doesn't grow in the mother's tummy or stomach! My goodness, kids say this all the time—that a baby is growing in the stomach—and we virtually never correct them. Well, from now on you will, okay? "The baby grows in the uterus, honey, not the stomach. The uterus is an organ made mostly of muscle; it's the size of my fist and is inside the mother's body right about here" (place your fist against your lower abdomen). "It can expand to hold a baby as it grows."

By about age eight you will want to have defined for *both* girls and boys all the words for the private parts and genitals previously mentioned, including the fallopian tubes, clitoris, labia, nipples, scrotum, and pubic hair. You'll also want to delve into an explanation of sexual intercourse, oral sex, anal sex, menstruation, and nocturnal emissions, and provide periodic clarification of masturbation, erections, and abuse prevention (see chapter 8). And you have to prepare yourself to explain to your child those slang sex words you do not want him or her to say, including the sexual slang not specific to body parts. Let's explore those.

Use Your Words

I strongly disapprove when a child uses sexual slang, no matter what his or her age is. And although some parents would not admit to it in public, particularly the more permissive parents, deep down most are really put off when their kids use slang. Now, you may say in front of others, "Oh, what's in a word? What's the big deal if your kid says *fuck* once in a while?" You may say this, but don't you recoil from it, deep in your core? Do you ever draw a line in the sand with your child concerning his use of slang? Are you making a concerted effort to stop your child from using slang or do you ignore it?

Granted, slang is probably the least significant sexual problem experienced among young people, but it is also one of the earliest to develop. When compared to sexual abuse and assault, teen pregnancy, sexually transmitted infection, and HIV, a child using slang is a minuscule problem. But it could be the beginning of bigger sexual problems down the road. In the field of crime prevention, it is now believed that if a community doubles-down on the lesser crimes, the minor infractions and misdemeanors, that it has a significant effect on more severe crimes. A similar idea could be applied to sexual problems—ideally, our efforts to combat more serious sexual problems among young people may improve if we make a concerted effort early on to eliminate sexual slang from our lexicon.

How Low Can We Go?

I think that the bar for what is acceptable sexually in our society has dropped *way* too low. At some point we'll have to raise that bar. Yes, I understand that many of us may think lowering the bar is fine as long as no one gets hurt. But as the bar sinks lower, and we don't notice it, our kids are being hurt. I think we need to reflect seriously about this. For example, if we accept having sex without love are we likely to see more sexual harm? Are we likely to see more unwanted pregnancy? Are we likely to see greater spread of disease and HIV? If we allow our children to accept lyrics in songs that debase women are we likely to see more violence toward women? If we accept more and more explicit sexuality into our daily lives are we likely to see more sexualized young people? If we allow kids to think that all vaginas are *cunts* and all penises *pricks*, all women hoes, and sexual intercourse and making love is just *fucking*, what effect is this having on our children's sexuality and subsequent behavior?

At the risk of sounding too conservative, I say that by lowering the bar of acceptability on our children's use of sexual slang we may set ourselves up for more serious sexual problems later on. Not that I believe that all kids who use sexual slang are headed down the road toward disaster. Far from it! But there are those who will be. There are some kids who will grow up believing that some very serious sexual matters are nothing more than a game to be played, and they will end up hurting themselves or someone else. So we can start right now and begin to raise the bar again. We can do so by taking a stand on our children's use of sexual slang.

Our morality and values are at the heart of our sexuality. We all take a stand on what we believe is right and what is wrong, and I have chosen to believe that sexual slang is something that adults need to discourage in children and adolescents. Not addressing it early on only increases the chances that it will take on a life of its own. In my experience, boys are more prone to using sexual slang than girls, who tend to be a little more secretive or coy. But these days it seems that more girls are using sexual slang and behaving this way than ever before.

An Ounce of Prevention

Even if you think your child hasn't yet learned or been exposed to a particular slang word I still encourage you to discuss it with him. Better he hears your words of caution when learning the slang words than to learn them on his own without your guidance. I know of a lot of teens who don't use slang around their parents but let it flow like water when around their friends. You're better off approaching your children when they're young and setting boundaries and limits than to just let it go and not comment until some of these words creep into your child's or their peers' lexicon. And eight years of age is where I would begin making my concerted effort.

This assignment is a tough one, because you may in fact be teaching your children a slang word he may not have heard yet. But once you've said the word to your kid you will likely not have to say it again. Your focus will then be on periodically reminding your child that you do not accept slang usage. So you might say to your eight-year-old, "I'm going to share with you some words that some kids your age and older use that I disapprove of. These are words I hope you won't use. You know how we've spoken about sexual and private parts of the body, and the purpose of those parts. Well, some of these words have other names for them that I would not want you to ever use. For example, some people call a penis a *prick*, a vagina a *cunt*, the testicles *balls*. Sometimes some people call sexual intercourse *fucking*. As your Dad (or Mom), I simply hate it when I hear these words. People use these words for several reasons; sometimes to get people to laugh, sometimes because they want to hurt another person by calling him or her a name, and sometimes just because they think it's cool. I very much hope you don't use those words as you grow older."

You can go over other slang words, but there should not be any reason why you would have to repeat those words to your child once you've discussed them. You can periodically remind him of your expectations for using words and make sure to praise him for not using slang: "I just want to compliment you on not using slang language; Mommy is so proud of you for talking respectfully." And you can use teachable moments when you hear certain slang language used: "I just heard that boy use inappropriate language. It makes me very uncomfortable to hear those words. I'm really happy that you don't say those words." Making references to language that is and is not acceptable to you as the parent should go a long way toward shaping your child's behavior and preparing him for the onslaught of slang that he will hear as an adolescent.

What Those Parts Do

Knowledge is power, and if kids don't understand how their bodies work sexually, they are weak and vulnerable. If I don't know what part of the body makes eggs, I probably don't know when I ovulate, or for that matter what ovulation is. If I don't understand ovulation then I sure don't understand menstruation, and if I don't understand menstruation then I probably have no idea when I am most susceptible to pregnancy. If I have no idea that my penis leaks pre-ejaculate semen before I actually ejaculate, I could have a big problem one day. Think of all the changes that one's body goes through during puberty. If your child doesn't have a reasonable understanding of what those biological and emotional changes will be, there is a significant chance that she or he will experience some level of confusion at some point. And it all adds up pretty quickly. The less a child knows about her body and what to expect as she develops, the greater the risk of that confusion. And the greater her confusion, the greater the possibility that she will make poor decisions concerning her sexuality.

We can all relate to the challenges of puberty and adolescence—and the challenges that kids experience today are far more significant than the ones we faced growing up. I will delve into many of these challenges, and what we need to do to help our children negotiate them, a little later in the book. But the early development of a sexual vocabulary provides a firm grounding for young people to not only better understand their sexuality, but also develop a reverence and respect for it.

By providing your child with an accurate sexual vocabulary, you become more approachable on sexual matters. Many parents simply give their child an age-appropriate book on sex to look at and read. But when parents do this, the book becomes the source of sex education and the parent takes on the role of a bystander. If you do share a book or two with your child, you *still* have to be the primary sex educator. All this parenting stuff is hard work, and no one ever said it was going to be easy. So let's make the effort and do it right.

You're off to a great start with your little one, with the gift of a sound sex vocabulary and basic knowledge of the body parts. These will make your task easier as you introduce your kindergartner to the classic "birds and bees" information: sexual reproduction.

CHAPTER 6

Everything They Learn About Sex Needs to Start in Kindergarten

I remember being asked to come and speak to a first-grade class about human reproduction around the time of the Monica Lewinsky scandal in the late 1990s. The teacher had some animal babies that had been born in her classroom—perhaps hamsters or guinea pigs—and wanted me to make the bridge between animal and human reproduction.

I had done this many times before. It never ceases to amaze me how capable six-year-olds are of absorbing the basics of how life is created. By the time I've finished the talk with them, one-third have gleaned the basics, another third of them haven't fully comprehended all that I said, and the final third are simply bored. Occasionally some will ask how the sperm cell and egg cell get together, and I will segue into a brief description of how sperm comes out of the penis and into the woman's vagina, the opening between her legs. They get fairly uncomfortable at that point; some will start giggling, some will stare, wide eyed, and some will not be sure what to do next. But that's the way it is with six-year-olds. At least I know I've provided a factual foundation for additional learning.

On this particular day, however, a totally unexpected question arose during my discussion with this class. This one little boy raised his hand and asked me, "Dr. Fred, did the president really pull his pants down and have that lady kiss his privates?" *Wow*, I said to myself, *did I just get asked a question about oral sex by a six-year-old? Well*, I thought, *welcome to the sexualized world of young children.* So after I regained my composure, I looked around the classroom and it seemed as though every other little six-year-old head in the class was nodding affirmatively, bobbing up and down. And it didn't take long for all the other students in the class to start chatting, with some raising their hands and asking questions and making comments. "Yeah, Dr. Fred, I heard that too," shouted out another boy. "I heard that on TV," said one of the little girls. "That's really yucky, Dr. Fred," said another. *Oh, boy*, I said to myself. *This is not what I came here to discuss.*

I quickly thought, *What would I say if these were my own kids? What would I want them to hear, and is it something I can say to other parents' kids without getting fired?* I do know that I have to say something in such situations; ignoring what kids legitimately ask or say about sex is not the way to go. Whatever I say, it's got to have validity, be as developmentally appropriate as possible, and also include some values or moral message. You know already that I'm a big believer in combining sexual information with some underlying values or moral message, so if I do try to respond it has to put the sexual behavior of oral sex into a values context.

If I had thought that that student was the only one who had the question about oral sex, I probably would have referred him to his parents to ask the question and avoided having the entire class hear my response. But I was certain that virtually every child in the class had heard something about the alleged episode in the White House. I'd like you to think about that for a moment. Thinking back to that time, there was literally nonstop news coverage about oral sex. Of all the TV-watching young kids in the country, how many had an adult help them make sense of what they were hearing? Perhaps not very many. As a result of this episode, there was also a secondary message being sent out that perhaps oral sex was not really sex. How much of an impact was that message having on young kids and teenagers at the time? We can only imagine what this was adding to children's sexualized wall of messages.

But getting back to that first-grade class, here's what I said: "Wow, you heard that too? Well, you know, kids, as strange and as weird as it sounds, there are some adults who love each other who will do that." "Oh, Dr. Fred, that's disgusting," could be heard among the many "oohs" and "ahhs" after I had said it. But within a few moments all quieted down and we moved on. As you can see, six-year-olds don't actually want to hear very much about sex; they just want their questions answered and their curiosity quelled.

Talk about a teachable moment! It may not have been the perfect answer, but to this day I can't think of a better one. I didn't ignore the question but acknowledged what the students had heard, I put the behavior of oral sex into an adult context where it certainly belongs, and I attached the values message of love to it. I may have stretched the truth somewhat in implying that love was involved, but, as I've said before, we want our kids to grow up believing that you should love, trust, and respect someone if you're going to put your mouth on a person's penis or vulva.

In a recent talk to a group of kindergarten parents, I made the following statement: "In just five very short years there is about a 50 percent chance that your little one will start puberty. And do you know that here in New York City almost 9 percent of kids have sex before reaching age thirteen?"[1]

(For those of you living elsewhere in the States, don't go thinking you're off the hook. Alabama and Arkansas, you're about 10 percent; Delaware, you're almost 10 percent; Mississippi, you're over 13 percent; and Dallas, Detroit, and Memphis, you're all higher than New York City.)[2]

"So in just a few years you're going to be confronted with some pretty difficult issues with your child, and that includes talking about when, with whom, and under what conditions you believe someone should have sexual intercourse. You'll need to discuss all the other types of sex as well!"

The kindergarten parents looked at me like I was from another planet. They stared at me with the most incredulous looks on their faces, and the room was so quiet you could hear a pin drop. "So if there's about an 8 to 10 percent chance that your child could be sexually active before age thirteen," I continued, "doesn't it make sense that you should be having some very serious discussions about sexual intercourse a couple of years before then? If 5 to 7.5 million U.S. kids are sexually active before thirteen, our serious discussions must start by ten years of age. And if we should be having serious discussions by age ten, shouldn't we have initiated some conversation about sexual intercourse a good deal before then? Is it out of the question, then, that by age eight we should be starting to discuss with our kid, with some regularity, what our expectations are for our kids with regard to sexual intercourse? This would mean that we should be sharing our views on the sanctity of the act, the risks and benefits of intercourse, and our values concerning when, with whom, and under what conditions intercourse should take place. All of this brings us to about age five or six, when we might have our first discussion of what sexual intercourse is. You can wait until eight years of age, but I'm telling you there is no harm in starting at five or six years of age. There are only benefits."

As you can see, I have allowed a several-year window for you to begin conversations with your child about sexual intercourse. This is deliberate on my part. While it is essential to have had some introductory discussions about sperm cells and egg cells and how they create a new life when joined together, I do not think it is essential to define sexual intercourse at five, six, or even seven years of age—but it is by age eight. However, as I've said, your child may ask you questions prior to age eight that lead you to initiate a talk in which you define intercourse. I also want you to understand that you can choose to bring it up yourself, and I will discuss how to do this. Doing so will obviously give you a head start, and please understand that there is nothing to worry about should you decide to initiate a talk at five or six. But you should realize that by age eight, it absolutely becomes relevant to start some serious discussion about sexual intercourse.

Returning to my talk that day with the kindergarten parents, I could feel the comfort level dropping in the room as some of the parents started squirming in their seats, looking around for some reaction from the others.

"If we discuss sex with them, can't that actually sexualize them?" asked a father. "Isn't there a chance that it could actually increase their interest in sexual matters?" he continued.

I get this question all the time, from parents of children of all different ages. I suppose that if your sex talks are preachy and bossy, or your talks are void of any sense of involvement or con- nection with your child, then you can expect no positive returns and possibly even some negative ones. But combine your talks with authenticity, empathy, dignity, and a real sense of bonding, and they will not increase a child's sexual behavior. They will, how- ever, increase your child's chances of delaying sexual involvement and help him or her to make better decisions about sexuality.

What Are We Really Afraid Of?

When our children are infants, most of us really don't think much about what we're going to say to them about sex when they get older. For the most part it's not on our radar screen yet, and even if it is, it's so far off in the future that we have a whole lot of time to prepare for it, right? And even when our children reach five years of age, we're still not really thinking too much about it. Sound familiar? But if you stop and think about children's development today and when puberty begins, a five-year-old is not that far away from having to manage some pretty heavy-duty sexual stuff. If the mean ages for menstruation and sperm development are in the eleven to twelve-and-a-half age range, and the initial changes of pubertal development frequently occur before then, sometimes as young as seven and eight years, then in reality there are large numbers of fairly young kids who are developing sexually and are actually capable of producing babies themselves. So a five-year-old is only a few years away from some big-time changes.

Let's face it: every five-year-old on the planet has probably asked, "How does the baby get into your tummy, Mommy?" As I've said several times before, your five- or six-year-old child is likely to be satisfied with an explanation of a sperm cell and an egg cell joining together and won't ask about how the sperm actually gets to the egg. But you need to be prepared if she does. And in that case, telling her the basic information will cause no harm.

It's No Dissertation

As I've already said a number of times, your five- or six-year-old doesn't have a whole lot of focused energy for learning about sperm, eggs, or how they get together. When you do have your discussion, it's all really rather quick. It's certainly no dissertation. As I wrote in the last chapter, by this point in your child's development you've laid the groundwork with the vocabulary, the names for the genitals and sexual parts. You've explained the testicles and the ovaries, and how the testicles make sperm cells and the ovaries make egg cells and how cells are very, very small. Making the bridge between the sperm and the egg is simple: "Daddy and Mommy lie in their bed without clothes on, and Daddy puts his penis into Mommy's vagina. The sperm come out of Daddy's penis into Mommy's vagina, and if Mommy's ovaries have made an egg cell, then a sperm cell can join together to make a baby." And as my favorite cartoons used to say, "That's all, folks."

Do not be concerned that you have only made reference to procreational sex and not made any reference to recreational sex. There will be plenty of time for that as your child gets a little older. You'll also have time later to explain how two moms or two fathers can have a baby, and you'll discuss adoption, single parent families, and the whole shebang as time goes along.

Of course, single parents and gay and lesbian parents will want to have that discussion right about now. However you had your child, you will want to, in a matter-of-fact way, let your child know how it happened. Here's one example: "Mommy adopted you. That means another man and woman made you. They could not raise you and that is when Mommy got you. Mommy wanted you as her baby and I couldn't love you any more than I do." I'm sure you'll have so many more talks, but the best time to tell your child how he was adopted is generally when you have the sperm and egg discussion. Gay and lesbian parents will do the same, explaining their particular situation of how they became parents.

Regardless of the family's individual circumstances and irrespective of family makeup, our five- or six-year-olds will handle these talks very well. Most all will cringe when the penis-in-vagina part comes but they'll manage all of this in good fashion. The only question is *will you?*

It's Never Too Early

Don't ever forget: it's never too early, but it can be too late! What I want you to do as you move forward with your five- or six-year-old is to periodically feed her little bits of information, personal values, and guidance about different aspects of sex and sexuality. There's no particular "flow" to follow when sharing with your child your wisdom on sexual matters. You certainly will not talk about sex every day, or even every week. Sometimes it will come up more often and other times you will have what seem like long dry spells. When a teachable moment presents itself, however, you should try to take advantage of it. They usually occur without any warning, but with all the different sexual messages that our kids receive every day there are more than enough opportunities for you to pick and choose the ones you will comment on with your child. Your formally planned talks will probably occur several times a year, possibly more, and will focus on information that you believe your child should learn.

I mentioned earlier that it takes time to become a good driver. Simply because you have passed your driver's license test in no way implies that you are a truly safe driver. It just means you have demonstrated an ability to drive. A teenager may be ready for some driving around on her own, but it takes years before she is really ready to face all the dangers of the road. Similarly, when a child enters adolescence, she or he is capable of sexual intercourse and pregnancy. Yet the adolescent is not ready for either. Perhaps the worst time to start a discussion of sexual intercourse and pregnancy is when your kid is a teenager. It's not the best time to expect them to start connecting with you on the subject; after all, the teenager's job seems to be to make our lives miserable, not to willingly do as we say with regard to their behavior. Decisions that have as much life-changing impact as sexual intercourse should not receive their first attention when one is in the throes of the biological and emotional upheavals that come with adolescence. Like I always tell parents, you don't want your fifteen-year-old kid to start to think about how far to go when she's already sitting on that park bench with that gorgeous boy who has a hand on her mid-thigh and is kissing her passionately. *Oops*, you're going to say, *I should already have had some discussion with her about that.*

The list of possible topics or issues that could be addressed with your five- or six-year-old can be quite extensive. Through your teaching, your child is learning vocabulary and functions of the body, various gender roles played out by boys and girls and men and women, safety issues, masturbation, sexual intercourse (depending on the child's readiness), and your values about many aspects of sexuality. They are learning by watching us as well—how we show love and affection, agree and disagree, solve differences, act as men and women, behave as husbands, wives, and partners. So much of what they will learn about sex and sexuality will really begin to take shape during the kindergarten and first-grade years. The building blocks for your child's sexual future truly start now.

So now is the time to begin to address some topics that will come up a few years down the road when your child must confront some very important decisions about sex. Learning about sexual intercourse, determining the type of person to be sexual with, and being able to postpone pregnancy until adulthood should not suddenly begin when these issues become relevant in a child's life. As I have said before, these are decisions of such magnitude that our children need to be learning about these issues long before they are faced with them.

As you scaffold your discussions about how babies are made, you will be discussing the values that you want your child to adopt about sexual intercourse, pregnancy, and the type of person to enter into a relationship with many years down the road. You will have discussions of the big three—love, respect, and trust—and how they should play a major role in all decisions about sexual intercourse. If, for example, you are in the park with your five-year-old and you see a baby with its parent, you might say, in passing, "You know, sweetheart, a person should only think of having a baby when she is an adult. There are too many teenagers who become pregnant." You might add to this during another teachable moment when you say, "People must be in love before they have a baby. They have to be really sure that they are in love with each other." You will scaffold that with even more talks: "It takes a long time to know if you love someone. It takes a long time to know if you can trust someone." You will also be mindful of being authentic in the things you say about all this. When walking by several teenagers outside a middle school, you could say to your five-year-old, "Remember when we spoke about how only adults should have a baby? What then would you say to a teenager who wanted to have a baby?" Or, if you are watching TV and see a parent taking care of a baby you could say, "Do you think a teenager can handle the big responsibility of taking care of a baby and being a mother?"

"YOU CAN'T DO THE THING WITHOUT THE RING"

You may want to give your child the message that two people should be married before having sexual intercourse or having a baby. This is of course anyone's prerogative to advocate. I personally do not say this to my child with regard to sexual intercourse; I just think it is too unrealistic. If you're thirty-five years of age and not married yet, you can't have sex? Or, if my child is gay or lesbian then he or she could never have sex because gay marriage is illegal in most states. I believe that this is simply an indefensible position to take. As for insisting that one should only conceive a baby in the context of marriage, that would mean sending the unmarried straight to the alternative methods now used by those who have trouble conceiving through intercourse but want to have a biological child—artificial insemination, in vitro, and surrogacy (also used by gays and lesbians, who obviously can't both produce their own biological offspring as a couple, and still can't get married in most states). Even without restricting sex to marriage, there is much to tell our children concerning when and under what conditions you expect them to experience sexual intercourse.

I'm sure as you read this some of you are probably thinking, *No way am I gonna do this.* That is because reading about doing this is probably stranger than actually having the conversation with your child. Children this age will handle what you are saying in a very matter-of-fact way. They will respond accordingly and then will want to move on to something different. Again, you are trying to share the values you want your child to learn in conjunction with sexual intercourse and having a baby. You want to instill in your child both the knowledge and the moral guideposts very early, and you will have these discussions with your child as you see fit over the course of the next several years. By doing this you can assure yourself that, by the time your child reaches adolescence, she or he will have a strong foundation upon which to make critical decisions about sex and sexuality. And you will have established a significant line of communication so that, as your child enters that stage of adolescent development where he naturally begins to pull back from you, there will still be a significant attachment that will make you very approachable.

Who Is Your Ideal Partner?

It is important to help your child develop a good understanding of the type of person he or she may want to develop a relationship with as an adult. Yes, age five or six is a long way from choosing a life partner, but getting the basic ingredients out early can only serve your child well. Once you discuss with your child the sort of partner that would serve one well, you can use those qualities as a reference point as your child eventually enters adolescence and young adulthood.

Whoever your present partner is (if you have one) will go a long way in teaching your child the sort of person you feel is worthy of an intimate and loving relationship. So if your partner, spouse, or life partner does not measure up, or maybe falls short of your ideal, then you need to realize this person likely stands as a negative model for your child. I've met far too many parents who have such a partner, and they wonder why their kids are having problems. If you have multiple partners in your life, you need to be especially careful regarding how this affects your child. (In particular, having multiple partners coming and going in your home is a potentially volatile and problematic scenario on a number of fronts.) Our kids watch us like hawks—the way we dress, the way we talk, the way we love, fight, argue, and show affection. If we show malice, disrespect, and nastiness, our child will be there taking it all in.

The most powerful way of teaching your child what sort of person she or he should consider as a partner, down the road, is to model on a day-to-day basis the human qualities you want your child to revere most. You and your partner have a huge responsibility regardless of whatever you say to or teach your child. So sketch out the values you want your child to embrace—such as empathy, love, respect, trust, responsibility, and honesty—and ensure that you incorporate them into your way of life. If you can model them regularly there is a far better chance your child will learn to embrace them in hers. Remember, the apple does not fall far from the tree.

Behavior: The Golden Rule

When teaching values, you'll take the same approach as you will in teaching your child about intercourse and pregnancy. You are always laying out the basics and then scaffolding your message as you move forward with your child. So you might say, "Some of the most important things you will ever learn in life concern how you treat other people. Learning to show respect to others is something that we all need to do. You need to try to understand the needs of others, what other people need in order to feel good and be happy, and what makes them sad and hurt."

When your child displays a behavior that is problematic, highlight the behavior for the child and tell him how it makes you feel, and how it might make others feel: "When I see you make fun of that child, it makes me feel sad. I bet it also hurts her feelings." When you do this you are helping your child learn empathy. And remember to always be authentic: "If you were a mommy and your child stole from another child, what would you say to her?" Or you might role-play a situation in which a child is trying to get your child to steal money from an open pocketbook in order to highlight how to say no and what the best course of action would be for handling such a situation. As you help your child understand the importance of certain basic core values, you are also helping him to appreciate the importance of developing relationships with persons who also possess those values.

TOO YOUNG FOR SEXY

Are you teaching your child to have an adult appearance? How are you dressing her or him? Does your little girl wear any makeup yet? Are you dressing her a little sexy sometimes? If her ears are pierced, are the earrings a little too extravagant at times? How about your son? Do you have an earring in him yet?

Then there are the hairstyles. Are you trying out wild looks on your kindergartner? Did you highlight her hair yet? You didn't give your boy a Mohawk, did you?

Is your little boy's baseball cap tilted to the side or turned around backward? Are his pants hanging on his hips? Does he act macho and tough?

Are you attempting to have your little girl look just like a runway model? Is she learning that sexy is better?

This is just some stuff I want you to think about.

Tell your child about the various qualities you look for in persons you want to be your friends, associates, and partners. Do this as often as you see fit to do. Comment on the positive and negative qualities of people you encounter in your lives. There will be times when you are watching TV or reading a book with your child and you will be able to comment on the character's behaviors, traits, and personalities. Planning your strategies for teaching your child what to look for and value in others will pay big dividends down the road as your child grows older. This lesson is as important as anything your child will ever learn in life.

While you're talking with your kids about the kinds of people who make good friends and partners, and how to treat others kindly and respectfully, you should also introduce the idea of sexual orientation. Let's talk about introducing this important subject to your kids.

Gays and Lesbians

When my son was five we had a couple of friends who were lesbians. I can remember very well when I decided to share with him that they were in love with each other. I simply chose a time when we were discussing them and I explained their relationship in a very matter-of-fact way: "Susan and Rhonda are lesbians. That means that they love each other like mom and dad do." My son looked at me and said, "Okay," and that was it. I later explained to him that two men can also love each other like Mom and Dad and Susan and Rhonda. I built on this awareness gradually, and within several months explained that gays and lesbians have sex with each other kind of like Mom and Dad have sex. A year or so later I remember having a discussion with him about how some people don't like homosexuals, and how there are people who bully them and try to physically hurt them simply because they are gay and lesbian.

We discussed how wrong that is—how no one should ever be harmed because of whom they fall in love with or want to have sex with. My son managed this information like any other six-year-old would, with a considerable level of concern for the safety of others.

When I go into a fifth-grade class and mention homosexuality, students giggle, groan, make faces, and roll their eyes. I can't help but think how we should all be beyond this by now. But with so many legal barriers still preventing full civil rights for homosexuals, and so much overt hatred and violence in evidence, clearly we still have a long way to go. I can imagine there will always be one or two students who have trouble accepting the reality of homosexuality, but closed-mindedness still seems to be in the majority with ten-year-olds. This tells me there is one of two possibilities at play. Either a majority of parents are teaching their children not to accept homosexuality, or a majority of parents simply don't talk about it with their kids and the kids are just reacting to something they perceive as different. I would prefer to think it is the latter of the two.

During one of my discussions with a fourth-grade class, I was talking about how two men or two women can love each other like a man and a woman can. I spoke about the need for tolerance and how many people who are perceived to be gay or lesbian are killed in this country every year. As I spoke, one of the students started to cry. This little girl said she has two fathers and that one of them had recently been beaten and hospitalized simply because he was gay. She confided that this was the first time any teacher had ever brought up the topic of homosexuality, much less how we should all be tolerant of gays and lesbians. She thanked me profusely for doing something that all teachers should be doing: discussing the reality that discrimination in this country also includes gays and lesbians. I have never forgotten that young girl.

We have covered just about every major sexuality topic that you should start talking about with your kindergartner, with one exception: masturbation. Because it will probably be your child's very first sexual experience, and because there is still so much misinformation, embarrassment, and secrecy attached to the subject, I decided that masturbation deserves a full chapter of its own. That chapter follows.

CHAPTER 7

No One's Ever Died from Masturbating

I suppose that once little children find their genitals, they never forget where they are. Young kids love to touch them, stroke them, pull on them, and rub them. They don't care much about the whole public and private behavior thing; all they really care about is that touching their genitals feels good and is very comforting. Little boys will likely begin to masturbate earlier than girls, simply because their genitals are easier to find—given that a boy's are outside the body and a girl's are inside. But by age five the girls do catch up.

Infants have the ability to orgasm, but more often than not masturbation serves more of a comforting function. We should regard masturbation as virtually universal in nature, occurring in all societies throughout the world. By now all of the problems previously associated with masturbation have been sufficiently debunked; very few problems are associated with it (except if it is done in public and/or done to excess at the expense of other activities of daily living). In fact, we now know that masturbation provides a number of positive benefits to children and adolescents. It helps the young child to learn about his or her sexual response, helps to relieve stress and anxiety, has been associated with a heightened self-concept and self-esteem, and of course helps to sharpen eye-hand coordination.

When Parents Disapprove

Growing up in a very devout Baptist household, I learned early on that the less I touched my penis, the better off I would be. It was something I just wasn't supposed to do. My father would admonish me if I touched it through my pants, my preacher and the church-going elders told me to never waste my seed, and even my older brother warned me about touching my penis too much. Needless to say, I had a lot of people warning me about something that all of my regular friends seemed to do a lot of: play with their penises pretty much as often as they could.

Even though the disapproval from the adults in my life couldn't be ignored, in the end masturbation prevailed. So on one particular evening, there I was, in my bed under the covers, the lights off, a flashlight in my right hand, nudie magazines spread out all around me, propped up on my right elbow and masturbating. Suddenly and without warning, the covers were pulled off and my father was staring down at me with a frown worthy of any criminal caught in the act of something terrible. "Look at what you're doing," he growled at me. Then he collected all the nudie magazines, said "This could get you into Hell," and stomped back to his bedroom to put the magazines back into his dresser drawer where I had found them.

Eventually I was able to look back and laugh at his reaction. But I'm sad to say that this is not just a hilarious story about a quaint attitude of yesteryear. To this day, there are parents who have a tremendous amount of difficulty accepting the fact that their kid masturbates. When I give presentations there are always a fair number of parents who either frown on their child's masturbation or would prefer they not do it as much as they do. I always share with them my experience with my dad, hoping to give them some insight into the futility of their efforts to get their children to stop. I share with them the considerable amount of guilt and angst that I experienced with my dad and how it stayed with me all throughout my adolescence. I can imagine, however, how hard it must be for those parents who feel as my dad did, experiencing that frustration of dealing with a child who is determined to do something that they don't want him to do.

Unfortunately for the children of parents who find masturbation unacceptable, their position can pose quite a challenge. The child can't resist doing it, and the parents spend a lot of time and energy trying to extinguish the behavior. But ultimately the parents will lose simply because masturbation feels too darn good to resist. Sadly, as many of these children continue to masturbate, they become increasingly consumed with guilt because they know their parents disapprove of it.

Contrary to what you might think, masturbation helps to reduce tension and relieve stress, and it helps the young adolescent to better understand his or her sexual responsiveness and preferences. In other words, it helps the child to recognize the sort of sexual excitation that gradually builds as one gets closer and closer to orgasm. It helps children understand what sorts of pressure, speed, and friction are needed in order to stimulate their genitals and cause orgasm. They can engage in it when they feel the need for sexual release, they don't need a partner to feel sexual pleasure, and, most important, it is very safe—indeed, it is virtually risk free. There is no risk of contracting an infection or disease and no risk of pregnancy.

THERE'S A TIME AND A PLACE

Kids need to hear the message from us that masturbation is a normal and positive part of life. But kids are *not* helped by parents on the other end of the spectrum who place no restrictions whatsoever on this behavior. Their message is, *Just go right to it, as often as you like*, almost anywhere or any place, as long as you don't interfere with other people. The problem with that strategy is that it's *not* always okay at any time or in any place. Not only are some of those places public, like our living rooms, but we simply cannot spend our time masturbating when we have responsibilities. While there might be times we'd rather stay home from work, hang out, and pleasure ourselves, we obviously can't do that, as we have more important matters to take care of.

So if you are a parent who doesn't want your kids masturbating, you've got to back off. Cut your children some slack. If you really can't come to terms with the reality that your child enjoys masturbation, at least tone down the disapproval level. Say something like, "You know I don't approve of your masturbation but I also understand why you enjoy doing it. I'm going to try to understand but I need you to also understand that it is against my beliefs. Still, I know it must be difficult to stop." I guess there really is no perfect response to give if you truly disapprove of the act of masturbation. You need to appreciate, however, that nothing you do will get your kid to stop.

Practice, Practice, Practice

It's important to realize that kids learn to masturbate in much the same way they learn how to drive a car or cross the street (but without you by their side as they practice!). It is a skill that needs to be learned, and it takes some time and practice to figure it all out. When we add psychological roadblocks to the mix—religious and cultural guilt and outdated fears such as "you'll run out of sperm"—we just make it all the more difficult for our child.

So we want to start out on the right foot by sending our child affirming messages about masturbation. More than likely, the first time you'll do this will be through a teachable moment. My guess is you'll have a whole bunch of teachable moments when it comes to masturbation and your child. That is, you'll probably "catch" your child touching, rubbing, and holding his or her genitals a number of times and at various ages. Perhaps the very first time you'll see your child touching his or her genitals will be in infancy, particularly with a boy. You are changing his diaper and your little one starts to play with his penis, which is then followed by an erection. By letting him do it and not moving his hand away, you send one of the earliest affirming messages he will receive about touching his penis and masturbation. You may well have a similar circumstance with your daughter, or perhaps it'll happen when she's lying on her stomach and grinding her pelvis into the mattress, or when she is humping her favorite stuffed bear.

And as kids get older and have developed some language skills, when we "catch" them we'll be able to verbalize our affirmation as well as broach the issue of privacy: "I see you touching and rubbing your penis (or vulva). When you do that it is called masturbation. I imagine that it feels good and Mommy and Daddy don't mind when you do it. But you need to know that it is a private behavior and you should do it in a private place like your bedroom." (A little note on what I have just suggested: you should notice that I said *vulva* and not *clitoris*. While the clitoris may be a primary body part that is stimulated by women when they masturbate, we do not believe that little girls use it in the same way when they masturbate. Typically we see a more general sort of rubbing against the vulva, perhaps because it simply takes time for young girls to identify where their clitoris is.)

We've known for some time now that masturbation actually occurs in utero. We are able to see little male and females fetuses touching and rubbing their genitalia while in their mother's womb. And all of us parents know that shortly after birth it isn't long before our little ones once again become reacquainted with their genitals. Kids' genital explorations are frequently random in nature and provide a pleasurable and calming response for toddlers. Gradually, over time, we begin to see a more purposeful attempt at stimulation. At exactly what age we begin to see a transition from random touching and exploration to a more purposeful attempt to stimulate the genitals is hard to say. We don't have a whole lot of empirical data to go by, but we might think of it this way. During infancy and throughout the first seven or eight years of life, the behavior is not true masturbation. As genital stimulation becomes increasingly more purposeful, and the child is actively seeking sexual pleasure, the behavior becomes more masturbatory. Certainly when puberty begins and the child progresses into adolescence and gains knowledge, we can safely suggest that the behavior becomes truly sexual in nature and it can be defined as masturbation. Fantasy begins to be included in the masturbatory activity, and the child usually starts to associate distinctly sexual images during his or her masturbatory episodes.

We also know that some boys, during early adolescence, will masturbate together with their peers. There are girls who will do this as well, but we believe that significantly more boys engage in mutual masturbation than their female counterparts. When masturbation is done mutually it should not necessarily be viewed as an indication that the participants are gay or lesbian. It is fairly common for both boys and girls to engage in some sort of same-sex behavior during adolescence, irrespective of whether they are straight or gay. When you think of kids entering adolescence and the significant awakening of sexual feelings and emotions that occur at this time, it makes total sense that certain young people will have some initial sexual interaction with those peers they are closest to. And young adolescents are typically closest to other kids of the same gender. Think of it as a kind of rehearsal for later sexual involvement. As these new sexual feelings emerge some adolescents will quite naturally act upon these feelings with members of their same-sex peer group. So we can probably safely say that some kids learn how to masturbate from observing and learning from their peers.

TRIAL AND ERROR

Most children learn how to masturbate on their own, just by trial and error. A rub here, a stroke there, a yank and a pull by the hand, humping or grinding the floor or a stuffed toy, slow, then fast, and faster—they find their own particular style, technique, and rhythm. It's not unusual, however, to refine one's technique as time goes along. My guess is that most kids learn through personal trial and error what works best for them.

Yes, You Can Teach Them This Too

Regardless of how a child learns to masturbate, as parents we should be ready and able to give some instruction to our children about how to do it. It doesn't have to be a lengthy or particularly detailed discussion of how to masturbate, but it can be several small conversations about certain techniques.

I am all in favor of suggesting, by the time your child is age eight or nine, that we weave in some mention of technique. For example, you might say, "You remember how Mommy has spoken to you about masturbation? That I think it is fine to do but that it is a private behavior? Well, there are certain ways to masturbate that are perhaps better than others. I find that touching the clitoris and rubbing it with different speeds is a good way to masturbate." What's that you're saying? Do you think I'm a little loony for suggesting this, and you can't imagine saying something like this to your own daughter or son? I know it can be embarrassing, but if you stop and think about it for a moment it really isn't any different from teaching your child any other fairly important skill in life. We teach our kids how to eat, brush their teeth, dress themselves, wipe their anus, and blow their nose, so why not masturbation?

Don't worry that it will make them want to do it any more than they already do. If you're uncomfortable having this talk, practice your talks with your partner, or in front of a mirror, and make sure you say the sexual words over and over. All of this will help to increase your comfort. I'll have more to say on the comfort issue in a little bit.

As I sit here and write all this I am smiling to myself as I remember having a discussion with my son when he was nine years old, not about how to masturbate (I had already done that) but rather what he needed to do about cleaning up afterward (important practical information!). I knew he enjoyed playing with his penis on a fairly regular basis and puberty was just around the corner. And I was concerned that as he started to enter puberty he would begin to ejaculate and I wanted to make sure that he didn't use his pajama bottoms or the bed sheet to wipe up his semen. As he enters puberty, even before a boy can make sperm or semen, he will emit a clear fluid from his penis when he masturbates.

"You know, you're going to enter puberty pretty soon and your testicles are going to start to make fluid, sperm, and semen," I said. "So when you masturbate you're going to have all that fluid come out of your penis. When you do start making that fluid, the first few times you will see that it is clear, and then eventually it will be a milky white color. About a teaspoonful will come out and it will be kind of gooey. You're going to have to capture it in tissues because I sure don't want you to use your bed sheet, or your PJs, or some other clothing."

His reaction was basically, "Yeah, okay, Dad."

By around age twelve I started to notice that puberty was beginning so I went through my little talk with him again.

"Yeah, yeah, Dad, I know, everything's good," he replied.

"Okay, son, I just want to make sure you know."

Well, as time went along, I would look for the telltale signs—a lot of tissues or toilet paper being used up, or any stains on the bed sheets. All of that was really quite silly on my part, but on a few occasions over the next several years I would kid him about it when his Mom and I would talk to him about cleaning up his room. I would say, "Pick up this, pick up that," and then finish by saying, "And make sure there's no semen on your bed sheets!" He'd always just roll his eyes and smile. He's seventeen now, but I still kid him that I don't want to see semen on the sheets.

I think it's great for a dad to talk to the son and for a mom to talk to the daughter initially about the masturbation process. But I also see no reason why the opposite gender parent can't make a comment or two along the way, as unprecedented or controversial as that may sound. So long as the conversation stays matter-of-fact, neither joking nor inappropriate, I think it's fine. This type of conversation is the reality for many single parents and gay or lesbian parents. If you are a single parent or gay and lesbian parent who finds yourself in the position of being the opposite gender of your child, I urge you to try to find a trusted, open-minded adult confidant of the same gender as your child to have periodic discussions about masturbation as well as other aspects of sex and sexuality with your child. If your younger child has a significantly older, same-gender sibling, avoid using him or her to teach the younger one, because the older child might tease or not approach the whole thing in the way an adult would.

How Much Is Too Much?

I've had my fair share of phone calls over the years from prekindergarten and kindergarten teachers concerned about students who were masturbating excessively. We see a lot of masturbatory behavior among this age group simply because many children this age have not learned sexual modesty and so they do it in public. Some of the calls are an overreaction on the teacher's part—they just don't want their students masturbating in class. But then there are those calls that present a student whose masturbation really is problematic. That is, the behavior occurs frequently, not only during rest times but even during classroom activities that should be keeping the students busy, including times when the entire class is working together. Many of these students stay actively engaged in the class activity but keep on masturbating.

When we see this sort of behavior it is often because the child isn't even aware of his or her masturbatory behavior. In all likelihood the child is masturbating simply because it is soothing and comforting but at the same time he or she is locked into the learning process and is not aware of the behavior. Sometimes we will see children doing it for just the opposite reasons. Because they are bored or not tuned into the learning process and the masturbation serves as a way to deal with that boredom.

The majority of students that I am called to consult on are masturbating in class for these two reasons, and when the behavior is brought to their attention it will usually stop in time. Of course, the teacher would alert the child's parents and solicit their support prior to speaking to the child. It is very important that the parents play a role in helping to extinguish the behavior. So the teacher might say to the student, "You are touching or rubbing your penis (or your vulva) in class. I know that feels good but the classroom is not the place to be doing that. If I see you doing it I will say your name and that will be the sign for you to stop." The parents can remind their child of the expected behavior each morning before school: "Now remember what we expect of you. You should not touch or rub your penis (or vulva) in the classroom." With the helpful reminders provided by the teacher and parents, along with any appropriate positive rewards, the child usually gains control of his or her behavior and the masturbation ceases.

When classroom masturbatory behavior is more difficult to extinguish, it usually occurs when the child is experiencing some sort of anguish in her life. There is something that is disturbing to the child; perhaps there is disharmony in the home or the child is in an abusive environment. The masturbatory behavior is serving as a way to release pent-up stress and anxiety or is a manifestation of an abusive event. In all likelihood a referral to an appropriate mental health provider would be required.

As your child grows older and enters puberty, masturbation becomes more sexual in nature, with the goal being orgasm. Many times I have stood in front of a class of ten-year-old fifth graders and spoken about masturbation and orgasm. Most of them know about masturbation. They may not know the term, but if I describe the behavior they know what I am talking about: "Masturbation is when a girl or a boy touches, rubs, or strokes their genitals or private parts in a way that makes them feel good."

Once, when I had to describe to the class what it is, one boy shouted out, "Oh yeah, Dr. Fred, choking the chicken" (another reminder for parents to teach proper names). But I can tell that most all of them know about masturbation by the look on their faces. Most of them break out in big smiles and then start whispering among themselves. Sometimes, if they ask, I'll get fairly specific as to exactly how one would masturbate: "A boy or man will usually stroke his penis up and down using different speeds; and a girl or woman will rub the area around her clitoris, which is very sensitive. Sometimes she'll go slow and other times will speed up." Admittedly, I often have to describe what the clitoris is by saying, "The clitoris is a part of a woman's body that is located just above the opening of her vagina. While most of the clitoris extends inside the woman's body, the part that she can actually see is called the glans and is on average the size of a pea. It is very sensitive when touched."

I will also lay out some boundaries and some values, to get them thinking on a personal level, by saying, "It is normal to masturbate and it is normal not to masturbate. Some people believe masturbation is perfectly fine to do, and some believe one should not do it. You should find the strength to have a discussion about masturbation with your parents, find out what their beliefs are about the behavior, and have them share their values about it with you."

Enter the Orgasm

When I discuss orgasm with kids, far fewer seem to have an understanding. While many ten-year-olds have likely had an orgasm, it's common for them not to appreciate what it was they actually experienced until they become more acquainted with it. As masturbation becomes more purposeful and deliberate, orgasm will follow and should become more plentiful. I generally define the term by stating, "An orgasm can occur if the boy or girl strokes or rubs his penis or her clitoris. An orgasm is an incredible feeling that originates in and around the genitals or private parts and lasts for about eight to ten seconds. And the feeling is really amazing." One time, a student raised his hand and asked, "But what is the feeling really like?" I thought for a moment and replied, "Well, you know what it feels like to have to sneeze and you can't? And you keep getting close to sneezing as you try again and again, but you still can't? And then finally your sneeze comes, and your whole body feels like it's exploding and it's all amazing? Well, that is kind of like an orgasm, only the orgasm is better, and it lasts a lot longer." I suppose there may be a better way to describe an orgasm but I've yet to come up with one. If you can think of one, please let me know.

Even when one engages in mutual masturbation the risk of harm to one's health is minimal compared to oral, vaginal, or anal sex. I believe it is totally appropriate to have a discussion about mutual masturbation with your ten-year-old daughter or son when discussing other forms of mutual sex behavior. When I do a risk-benefit analysis with students of the different forms of sexual interaction one can have, mutual masturbation always beats out the different forms of intercourse because it poses the least possible risk and harm. That is, if you are going to share sexual intimacy with another person, masturbation will get you into less trouble than any of the intercourse behaviors. Nevertheless, I always point out the one major risk from mutual masturbation, which is of course the turn-on factor. When it is done in an undisciplined manner, it can certainly lead to intercourse. One thing I always hear from teenagers who start out wanting to remain abstinent until adulthood but end up having sexual intercourse as a teen is that "one thing leads to another." Therefore, I also always discuss mutual masturbation in the same context as the different forms of intercourse—that is, that one needs to be an adult and have love, respect, and trust as a foundation to one's relationship with another before ever considering engaging in intimate sexual behavior.

Using Pornography and Fantasy

When people masturbate, many will usually use some sort of fantasy or set of images that provides a stimulus or turn-on effect. In short, they help us to reach orgasm quicker than we would without them. I bring this issue up because as parents we may need to be concerned with the sorts of sexual images our child is masturbating to. I want you to think for a moment about the possible effects that masturbating to certain images might have on people over time, particularly a young teen. If the images one masturbates to are devoid of a loving emotional component, portray women as objects, or incorporate violence or blatantly debasing forms of sexual interaction, what are the possible consequences over time? It doesn't matter whether these images come in the form of explicit visuals, as in video or pictures, or in the form of images we create in our minds through fantasy. The more one masturbates using these sorts of images the greater the likelihood that the behaviors depicted in them will become a source of sexual arousal. So if one masturbates to, say, a set of images that depict forced sex, then the behavior of forcing someone to have sex becomes sexually arousing.

Masturbating to sexually explicit images is likely to have a reinforcing effect, which can serve to condition a person to want to see more and more of the same images. As a person fantasizes the same images during subsequent masturbatory episodes, he will frequently put himself into the fantasy. In other words, he becomes a participant in his own fantasy. Obviously, the long-term concern is whether the person will at some point make his fantasy a reality. There have been very few studies of the effects of sexually explicit or pornographic images on young people. Studies with adult populations inform us that pornography is more like a fuel that gets put on a fire.[1] There is usually some predisposition already present that makes someone more prone to act a certain way, and the pornography becomes the trigger. For example, before committing a sexual offense, pedophiles will frequently "fuel" themselves by watching child porn.

I suppose the big issue for us as parents is how we should buffer our children from any possible negative side effects that could exist from viewing and fantasizing about certain sexually explicit images. I think most adults would agree that any prolonged watching of any sexually explicit material, especially material that does portray violence or images of debasement, can be potentially unhealthy for young people. Most parents would have a problem if their child masturbated to these sorts of images, whether by watching explicit material or by conjuring images through fantasy. None of us, for example, wants our kids turning on to thoughts or images of forced sex.

So exactly what should be our role in all of this? Well, I think we can screen and monitor our child's access to sexually explicit material for only so long. Through our vigilance we should be able to do a fairly good job up to and including our child's middle school years. Once our kids get into high school this becomes a little bit harder to do. You've already heard me discuss our roles in monitoring what our children are exposed to and how we can best help them to make sense of their sexualized wall of messages. This is no different. If we do what I have prescribed earlier in our attempts to be approachable, by the time they are older and do have access to pornography they will be able to deal with it responsibly.

So by age ten we should be having some discussion about the world of sexually explicit videos and pictures out there on the Internet, on cable and pay per view, and in print: "It's important that you understand that there are so many videos, movies, and pictures that show people having sex that are available over the Internet, TV, and in magazines. Dad (or Mom) believes that a lot of it is just garbage. They show a lot of men and women as being kind of sex crazed. What I mean by that is it makes them seem like they can't get enough sex, or they show men hurting women and taking advantage of them, or they show men and women having sex without love, and there are even movies that are pretty weird, showing things like people having sex with animals, or grown-ups having sex with kids. It's just garbage and we wouldn't want you to ever watch it."

I don't think you need to say much more than that at age ten. Probably the strongest buffer you can provide your child is through your parenting style. Being that authoritative parent is so important because you will be setting boundaries for your child regarding what is right and wrong, good and bad. As your child gets into middle school you will want to continue your discussion of sexually explicit and pornographic material. You will continue to reinforce your concerns for how these images distress you and you will also discuss how people will sometimes masturbate while looking at them: "I've spoken to you before about sexually explicit stuff on the Internet and in magazines that are out there. I hope you are not looking at any. So much of it is not what sex between people who love each other is really like." You can also mention fantasy during masturbation. You don't need to ask your child if he or she fantasizes during masturbation. Rather, you can make some remark that is more indirect but gets your point across: "If you think of sexy things when you masturbate, I hope it's not anything weird—you know, anything hurtful or dangerous." Leave it at that for now, but feel free to revisit the subject in little talks like these as time goes along.

Our talk about masturbation has led us to related subjects and brought us to the middle school years. Now we need to backtrack. The next chapter is all about preparing children for puberty and helping them through it. Your preparation phase starts with age eight and continues through ages nine and ten—reaching the threshold of middle school.

CHAPTER 8

Puberty: Preparing and Beginning Together

Is it possible that your child could actually start puberty at seven or eight years of age? It's kind of hard to believe, isn't it? Yet there is a growing concern that the development of secondary sex characteristics in girls, such as breast growth and pubic hair, is starting at increasingly earlier ages. Suggested causes range from environmental factors that involve hormonal influences to childhood obesity to the hypersexualization of young kids. While most experts believe that the age of onset of menses in girls and the development of sperm in boys have likely remained relatively unchanged over the past couple of decades, there are increasing concerns that secondary sex characteristics in girls are beginning earlier.[1] From a purely empirical standpoint, I think we really don't know what's going on out there, but it's probably pretty safe to say that some fundamental change is under way.

What is most important for us as parents, however, is to understand that we need to begin to have some serious discussions and conversations about the physical and emotional changes of puberty *before* our kids start these changes. So, because you don't know whether your child will start puberty at eight, nine, ten, eleven, or twelve years of age, I recommend that you start discussing it at eight; this way you'll be fairly certain of starting before puberty has begun. Before proceeding further, let me mention seven-year-olds briefly as I do not want you to think I'm avoiding that age group. I think of the seven-year-old as an "in-between" age. That is, we need to continue to reinforce with them what they have learned as six-year-olds, but they are still a little too young to be hearing what we will say to our eight-year-olds. However, be on guard. Should your child begin puberty as early as seven, you will of course have to begin addressing it.

We've talked about a whole bunch of important stuff up to now, and, if you've followed what I've laid out, you and your child are in an excellent position to have some big-time talks about the coming journey through puberty. From now until your child reaches young adulthood you need to make absolutely certain that you are the number one source of sexual guidance for your child, because things are really going to start heating up.

In this chapter I detail some of the information that I think is most important to highlight for your child as she or he prepares for and moves through puberty. It may seem like a lot, but I cut through the fat and lay out for you the critical pieces you'll want to focus on. I give you facts about puberty and sexual behavior in relationships, because you need to have a basic understanding of the physical changes that occur and some of the concerns your child will have about those changes—but I urge you to keep it simple. By no means do you have to be a walking, talking sexual-facts encyclopedia. This is not rocket science! You also need some understanding of how to help your child feel normal throughout puberty's duration, and a feel for the sort of peer pressure a child can expect and how to best deal with it. You need to know how to help your child use critical thinking to make responsible decisions, and how to help your child reflect on values that are life enhancing and enriching. This chapter will provide guidance on how to accomplish these tasks. I just don't want you to feel overwhelmed. Don't feel you have to go to the library or do research on the Internet on puberty and teen sexuality. I have aimed to provide what you need in this book. It's okay to feel embarrassed when you have these conversations with your child, but there are some basic things you can do to feel more comfortable. The more comfortable you are, the more effective your communication with your child can be.

I highlight some of the more important issues that I think require your use of authentic instruction—using actual life situations that involve sexuality to help your child better relate to what you want him to learn. There are many moments when you can choose to be authentic in your instruction, but there are some when you absolutely *must* be. Ultimately, your most effective tool for leading your child through the minefields of puberty and adolescence is your ability to communicate your values, consistently reinforce the boundaries of sexual behavior, and teach your child how to make good decisions about sex and sexuality. This chapter shows you how to package it all for your eight-year-old and then for your nine- and ten-year-old.

I repeat my earlier observation: we are a sex-stupid society. Most of us have had virtually no formal sexuality education or parenting education in our lives, yet we (and our parenting partner, if we have one) must be the number one sex educator for our children. I think it is much easier to get away with a minimal understanding of the body and how it functions sexually when our children are very young, but as they go through puberty and adolescence we have to kick it up a notch. There is absolutely no harm in having to tell your children that you don't have an answer to one of their questions but will find it out and get back to them; however, you must try to stay at least one step ahead of them in your knowledge of how the body functions sexually, especially during the latter part of elementary school and through middle school. By the time your kids are in high school they need less factual information from you, but of course will continue to need your moral and ethical guidance on how best to navigate their sexual world.

What Kids Really Need to Know About Puberty

So many of the concerns that kids have throughout puberty arise because they simply don't realize that the changes they are going through and the issues they are confronting are indeed normal. We adults can forget how difficult it is to go through puberty. There are so many developmental, psychological, emotional, and social changes going on that it can get overwhelming for our children. Any way we can help minimize our children's anxiety and stress will go a long way toward helping them manage these tumultuous years.

Kids at this age are prone to feeling like they stand out, almost like they have a scarlet letter on their chests, when they think they're different from others. It's likely that your child will frequently feel inadequate and out of place. He'll worry that whatever he's experiencing is only happening to him—that he'll be the only one at the party with a pimple on his forehead. Peer acceptance becomes even more important as a child progresses through adolescence. The more a child feels out of the norm, the harder the struggle for that acceptance. So expect to spend time just helping your child to feel normal.

Kids also have the major developmental task of negotiating newly discovered sexual feelings and urges. As parents, we need to remember not only the pulse-pounding, butterflies-in-the-stomach sensations we experienced from these new sexual feelings, but also the mixed bag of intense emotions—feeling confused, nervous, anxious, and scared—that often came along with the feelings. Let's face it: our journey through adolescence was a long, strange trip indeed. It is probably even more of a dramatic journey for young people today.

I have consistently found that if you establish yourself as an approachable parent prior to your child's puberty, the entire puberty and adolescent experience becomes far more manageable for your child and for you.

Look before you leap should be your motto. If you know what lies ahead, you will be better prepared when you get there. So you tell your daughter about menstruation *before* she comes to you with blood on her fingers. And you tell your son about wet dreams *before* he awakes one morning with semen stains in his PJs and on the sheets. And you help them to explore the sexual feelings they can expect to have for other kids when in middle and high school before they actually experience them for real.

So take out a pen and paper or turn on your computer and start to take some notes. What follows are the most important pieces of information and words of wisdom about puberty that I believe you need to know and share with your children, followed by commentary as needed. We'll get to more specific responses to these concerns in the following chapters.

Body hair, pubic hair, voice changes, sweating, oily skin, and pimples are some of the changes experienced by both genders. Breast development, widening and padding of the hips, and the ovulation and menstruation cycle are the unique changes for the girls; broadening of the shoulders, increased muscle mass, enlargement of the testicles, growth of the penis, and sperm/semen development are the unique changes for the boys.

When puberty begins. No one can predict when puberty will begin for any child. Some kids begin earlier, other kids later. Whenever it begins for your child is the right time. Also, no one can predict the particular order in which the various changes will occur. You should caution your child not to compare himself to his peers with regard to who started puberty first or who is developing faster or slower; every child's progression of puberty is different. If your child is either developing earlier than peers or lagging behind them, stay on guard for other kids who may be making fun of her or even bullying her. Being "overdeveloped" or "underdeveloped" makes a child an easy target for other kids. Keep your lines of communication open with your child and stay in touch with your child's teachers; you can also get a sense of how things are going by paying attention to how your child's friends are acting.

Body image. Even if your child appears to be progressing through puberty in a typical way, you should still be on guard for any disturbance in body image. Being concerned with how one looks is normal. But you don't want your child to become overly obsessed with thoughts about not measuring up to peers' (or the media's) standards; nor do you want the opposite—the child thinking he's so hot that he's just to die for. Start early to set the right tone on this issue with your child.

Hormones. Most of the physical changes of puberty occur because the body is producing more and different hormones than previously. These trigger changes in various body parts. Boys and girls actually share many of these hormones, just in different amounts.

Hair in new places. Both boys and girls will notice new hair growth. The amount and location of hair adults end up with varies widely among individuals, but one thing we all have in common is the pubic hair that grows around the genitals. Its purpose is to help keep that area of the body clean and to protect from chafing.

Perspiration. Puberty causes changes in the sweat glands; the increased perspiration, along with the growth of pubic and armpit hair, means that both boys and girls need to wash more frequently. They may want to start using deodorant, too.

Acne. In puberty there's an increase in facial oil, which helps to keep the face healthy. But if a child doesn't wash regularly (and sometimes even if she does), skin cells that shed from the face can mix with the facial oil to clog pores in the skin, causing the infections known as pimples or zits. Every adolescent will likely get some pimples.

Voice changes. Both boys and girls experience voice changes, but boys will experience a greater degree of change. It is common, when the voice is undergoing changes, for it to "crack." This can occur when a boy least expects it and can be embarrassing if it happens in front of a lot of people. The voice transition generally takes several years.

Breasts. Girls may be distressed to find that one breast is becoming slightly larger than the other. This is normal. In fact, there is some asymmetry in everyone's body; hands and feet are often slightly different sizes too. Media images, especially of women with breast implants, don't help us to have realistic expectations of our bodies. Breasts come in different shapes and sizes; they're all good breasts.

Nipples. Both girls' and boys' nipples can become hard, particularly when rubbed.

Penises come in all different sizes; they're all good penises. They are all big enough to do the job they were intended to do.

Circumcision. Most boys in the United States are circumcised. All boys are born with a sleeve or hood of skin called the *foreskin* covering the head of the penis. If parents choose to have their baby boy circumcised, in a procedure in which the foreskin is removed, it's done within a few days after birth. Boys who are not circumcised need to pull back the foreskin to clean underneath when they shower or bathe every day; otherwise bacteria can grow and cause an odor.

Testicle changes. One testicle will usually hang lower than the other. Sometimes when a boy is really anxious or feeling really cold, his penis can shrivel up somewhat and the scrotal sack that holds his testicles can as well. Sometimes the sack shrivels so much that his testicles seem to rise up toward his abdomen and almost disappear.

Erections. The penis becomes erect when more blood enters it than leaves it. A boy can have an erection many times during the day and can have them for no sex-related reason whatsoever. In fact, when least expected—boing!—an erection can occur. Tell your son that if this happens in front of people, just be cool and relax, and it will eventually go down.

Ovulation. Ovulation occurs when a mature egg cell emerges from an ovary. The egg cell lives for about twenty-four hours after ovulation. If not fertilized by a sperm cell, it dies and is flushed out through the vagina.

Women generally ovulate about twelve to fourteen days before the start of the next period. Most have no sensation associated with the event.

The uterine lining. Every month the uterus prepares itself for a pregnancy, creating a thick, blood-rich lining to support the implantation of a fertilized egg. If a sperm cell fertilizes the egg cell, it completes the journey down the fallopian tube to the uterus and burrows into the lining to receive nutrients as it develops into an embryo and then a fetus. However, most of the time the woman is not looking to become pregnant. If there is no fertilized egg cell, the uterus's lining is flushed out of the uterus through the vagina. This is called *menstruation* or *getting her period.*

Menstruation. When a girl first starts having menstrual periods it is fairly common for it to occur somewhat irregularly. She may skip a month, or at times she may have what appears to be two periods in one month. A menstrual period lasts about five or six days, during which about a half a cup of fluid flows from the uterus through the vagina. Most girls use a sanitary pad when they first start menstruating. As they grow older many will begin to use tampons. Menstrual periods and ovulation end sometime in a woman's fifties, on average, over a period of years called *menopause.* Many girls and women experience some discomfort when they menstruate. This usually involves some mild cramping, some feeling of bloating, and maybe a little moodiness beforehand. Should a girl experience any severe pain or discomfort she should inform her parents and they can consult their health care provider.

Wet dreams. It's common for boys to occasionally ejaculate while sleeping; that is, semen (a liquid that contains sperm cells) comes out of his penis. This is commonly called a *wet dream.* The boy does not necessarily have a sexy dream when this happens; he may simply ejaculate.

Masturbation is the term for the practice of stimulating one's own genitals to create pleasurable feelings, which may include orgasm (and, for boys, ejaculation). It's normal to masturbate, and it's normal not to;

it just depends on the individual. When a man ejaculates, the semen he releases through his penis contains 300 million or more sperm cells. He makes millions of new sperm daily and always has a considerable reserve of sperm within his testicles. He can never run out of sperm because of the number of times he masturbates. Even if a boy or man decided to masturbate several times every day this would only result in his semen containing less sperm. Sperm cells that are not ejaculated live in a man's body for about ten days and then die. When sperm cells die they are absorbed or discharged in the urine.

Sexual feelings. Perhaps the biggest change of puberty is the development of sexual feelings. For the first time your child will have to learn to respond to emotions triggered by sexual stimuli. Although children are capable of sexual response prior to puberty, this doesn't necessarily include an emotional response. Now it does. A significant developmental task for your child is to understand how to manage, control, and ultimately adjust to these newfound sexual feelings.

Starting to Talk About Puberty

Puberty includes all the physical and emotional changes that the body experiences when transitioning from a child to an adult. Puberty usually ends by the age of nineteen or twenty. Again, one of the most important things to tell your child right from the outset is that no matter when your body begins to change, whenever it does, it is the right time for her. The right time isn't when her friends start the changes of puberty or when her friends and peers say it is the right time. Whether she starts earlier, later, or about the same time as most others, her time is the right time.

I find that puberty talks with the nine- and ten-year-olds go over very well, with each group having a pretty keen interest in hearing about their expected bodily changes. Eight-year-olds need a much more abbreviated talk but will also show interest, with perhaps a little more trepidation.

When you begin your discussion, particularly with the nine- and ten-year-old, if you are somewhat shy about describing the changes that are more sexual in nature, then feel free to start with some of the more benign changes that occur. You start first with a little intro into hormones—chemicals produced by the body that cause many of the physical changes of puberty. You can then start a discussion about how the body begins to fill out and become more robust, or a conversation about how the body will begin to perspire more and how they must now wash and bathe more carefully than when they were younger or bacteria will remain on the body, causing body odor. Or you can begin with a talk about pimples and how washing the face with mild soap and water and patting it dry with a clean towel helps reduce the chances of developing the dreaded zits.

While all of this information about puberty is important for your child to learn, providing specific information about sexual behavior within a relationship is vital. Below are my suggestions for what you will want to convey to your child about sexual relationship behavior.

The Important Facts of Sexual Relationship Behavior

As you continue your puberty conversations you can start to weave in discussions of behavior within a sexual relationship, managing sexual feelings, and how to behave responsibly. I will offer ideas for doing that as we move along; for now, acquaint (or reacquaint) yourself with some of the important facts you will eventually share with your child.

- The risks of being sexually active as a teenager far outweigh the benefits. No matter how you look at it, engaging in intercourse before adulthood poses a significant risk of harm.

Unplanned pregnancy, sexually transmitted disease and HIV, abuse, and emotional regret from being sexually intimate and then experiencing a relationship breakup are very significant risks to a child's health and well-being.

- During sexual intercourse a man's penis will leak sperm and semen prior to ejaculation. One always needs to be aware of this. The idea that a man can pull out his penis before any sperm is released is not accurate. His penis is always leaking before he ejaculates.

- Most women ovulate about twelve to fourteen days prior to their next menstrual period. If a woman has sexual intercourse as she is ovulating she is more prone to becoming pregnant, if she and her partner are not using any form of contraception.

- Almost 39 percent of sexually active high school kids did not use a condom the last time they had sexual intercourse.[2] It's enough of a problem when teens have sexual intercourse at all. But to have sex and not use a condom is beyond stupid!

- Using a condom correctly along with another form of contraception is more effective at reducing the risk for pregnancy. Using contraception without a condom during sexual intercourse does not protect against HIV transmission.

- The only 100-percent-effective method of preventing pregnancy is not to have sexual intercourse. No form of contraception or birth control is more effective. None!

- Oral sex and anal sex are both sex. Whoever thinks they're not has another think coming. Teens need to understand that putting a mouth on a penis or vulva or a penis in the anus are indeed sex.

- When a woman starts becoming sexually excited it takes some time for her vagina to become aroused enough for sexual intercourse. Her vagina needs to lengthen and widen and it needs to lubricate or become wet. If a penis or some other object is inserted into her vagina prior to arousal it will likely be painful. A man on the other hand can be fully sexually aroused much quicker, literally within seconds.

- If someone has HIV in their body, the virus is found in significant amounts in that person's blood, semen, and vaginal fluids. This is why HIV can be transmitted through sexual intercourse, anal intercourse, and oral sex.

- The only 100-percent-effective way of preventing sexual transmission of HIV is to avoid sexual intercourse: vaginal, oral, and anal. If one has sexual intercourse, the only effective way to minimize the spread of HIV is to use a latex (rubber) condom (or vinyl condoms for those allergic to rubber). And even then it has to be worn responsibly—condoms can break and slip off the penis during intercourse. It must also be taken off the penis with care after ejaculation; otherwise semen can leak into his partner's body.

- Even if a teenager has had sexual intercourse they can still become abstinent. Previous sexual activity does not mean that one cannot become sexually inactive. Some teens think that once they've started they really can't go back to abstinence, but that's not true. It's never too late to stop having sex.

- Far more kids in middle school do not have sexual intercourse than those who do.

- More high school kids have not had sexual intercourse than those who have had it. (It is important to highlight this for our children. Many kids think most teens are having sex.)

- More than 10 percent of high school girls have been forced to have sexual intercourse. About 20 percent of girls who are in a relationship report physical or sexual violence in their relationship. Physical violence is just as high in teen homosexual relationships as it is in straight relationships. Kids need to hear this and think about how and why violence occurs so frequently in relationships.[3]

- Almost 22 percent of high school kids were high on alcohol or drugs the last time they had sexual intercourse.[4] It's very dangerous to have sex while intoxicated, because the ability to think clearly and act responsibly is diminished. We need to let our kids know how much we are concerned about their sexual behavior, as well as their alcohol and drug use, and that we are only focused on their well-being when we talk to them about these concerns.

You will begin to share some of these facts with your child when she turns eight years of age. Certainly by ten years of age you will want to have shared all of these facts as well as having started some authentic instruction around making good sexual decisions.

It Takes Practice to Get Comfortable

There is no better way for a parent to become more comfortable when discussing puberty related issues with your child than practice, practice and more practice. This is true of most things in life, isn't it? The same holds for when you talk about sex and sexuality with your child. The more you do it, the more comfortable you will become. And you don't necessarily need to have someone else to practice with. That's right, you can practice alone. Just take whatever it is you want to say to your child and say it to yourself. Create the scene in your mind and go right to it. You can also practice in front of a mirror; then you can get a feel for your words but you can simultaneously see how you look as you say it.

You can get a sense of the type of body language and hand gestures that you might want to use when you talk, as well. You can also videotape or audiotape yourself. I know this may seem a little extreme but you will want to do whatever it takes to get comfortable.

No matter how much you practice on your own you should make every effort to practice with someone else, too. Get your partner, your friend, or a relative—anyone who can give you some objective and reliable feedback and practice with them. It would be very helpful if this person could pretend to be your child and reply to what you are saying. Role-playing like this can be especially helpful, as it forces you to have to respond to the unexpected statements and actions the other person could pose to you. If taken seriously by the other person, this is a very effective way of practicing.

Of course, the best practice is to actually talk with your child. You can get some of the jitters out of the way by setting up your talks with your child beforehand. Before you actually get into the gist of your puberty conversations you can say, "You know, this isn't easy for me. My mom and dad never really talked with me about sex and I haven't had much practice. So bear with me. I may be nervous; I may not have all the answers to your questions. But I want to talk with you about this stuff because it is very, very important, and I love you, and I want you to be safe and to grow up happy and healthy. So hang in there as I talk. Listen carefully and please share with me your thoughts on what I say." Do what you need to do to establish your comfort level for your talks. Just giving yourself permission to admit to your child that this makes you uncomfortable may help immensely. But remember, the more you have these talks with your child, the more comfortable you will become.

Focus on Authentic Instruction

As I've mentioned before, using authentic instruction is a very effective way of helping your child learn how to think critically and make decisions that are healthy and wise. Of the many different issues about sex and sexuality where you can use authentic instruction, there are certain issues that absolutely require it. So heed what I recommend here, as you will want to become as proficient as you can in your use of authentic instruction with your child. Some of the choices and decisions your child makes about sex and sexuality will be some of the most important of her life. Authentic instruction will help her learn how to make the right ones. Here are the issues where you must use authentic instruction when working with your child.

Sexual Feelings and Decision Making

Most of our children will become sexually active when they become adults. Determining when and with whom is tough enough; being fully responsible is even tougher. Our children have a lot to think about and plan for to be ready for sex.

You will want to use plenty of authentic instruction when helping teach your child how to manage and negotiate sexual feelings. When your child learns how to do this he will be in a far better place for making good sexual decisions. Part of your task is to help him learn how to make decisions when he's confronted with intense sexual feelings.

Love, Respect, and Trust

As I've said at length already, when you have these in a relationship you just never have to worry about how your partner will treat you. Helping our children understand when these are present in a relationship is a major undertaking. I'll give you some examples later in this chapter.

Peer Pressure

When I work with a class of children on the challenge of saying no to one's peers, I find that many children are surprised to hear how hard it is for other kids to say no. Saying no can conjure intense feelings of being cast out of the group; it can seem that somehow it's the end of the world to have to say no to your peer group. When kids share their fears about saying no it helps them to know that other kids feel the same way. They come to appreciate that anyone who tries to get you to do something that is not healthy or good for you can't possibly be someone you should be friends with or hang out with. Understanding this will sustain them during some very difficult peer group moments.

As you will see, using authentic instruction will give your child the best chance to fully understand and integrate information, make better decisions and develop important communication skills, and develop an awareness of crucial values inherent in being a sexually responsible person.

Make Yourself an Approachable Parent for Your Child

The years from ages eight to ten are the time to solidify your identity as an approachable parent on all things sexual. Once your child leaves fifth grade and enters middle school, your child's peer group will become the one real threat to everything you've done right over the years. Yes, the media will be a factor, but the kids our children will associate with from middle school into high school can have a tremendous amount of influence on our children. It is essential that you know who your child's friends are and who his primary peer group is, and that you continually monitor their activities. If your child turns to a negative and deviant peer group, you are going to have your hands full, and more so if you are not keeping tabs on your child's social life. However, if your child has friends and peers that are thoughtful and nurturing, and if you have worked hard to ensure that you are an approachable parent, your child will have a far better transition into adolescence. This is why I urge you to talk so much with your child by ten years of age.

If you think the advice in this book has been a little over the top, or that the idea that ten is the new sixteen is stretching things a bit, all you have to do is hear from parents who have lost this battle and you will have a change of heart. Not only is it the right thing to do for your child, helping her transition as beautifully as possible into adolescence, but it will provide invaluable insulation from all the negative influences that can come with being a teenager. It is why I've highlighted the need to use authentic instruction when helping your child deal with peer pressure. Coming to terms with peer pressure is a major developmental task of adolescence.

Prepare to Weather the Changes— and Accept Them

The change from child to adult brings with it many different challenges, not just for the child but for his or her parents as well. Let's face it; it isn't easy going through puberty and it sure isn't easy to help your child as she goes through it. It is truly amazing how our children go from chatty, loving, adorable little human beings into these creatures who at times are barely recognizable. Puberty and adolescence have a way of making every parent on the planet ask the question, *What has happened to my darling little child?*

One thing is universal: the hormonally charged adolescent's job in life is to make his parent miserable. That is just the way it is; it's not because you're doing something wrong, necessarily—it is just the way of the teenager. Once you accept this fact and realize that it really isn't about you, you'll have eliminated a major roadblock as you move forward.

Too many of us parents get hung up on this reality. We just cannot understand what has happened to our kid and we expend a lot of energy trying to figure out how to get our sweet little child back. The big irony here is that we haven't lost our child at all; we only think that we have. Once we accept that she's still our daughter, just not our daughter the little child anymore, the quicker we can move on and establish ourselves as approachable to her in this new phase of her life. She is still our child but becoming a teenager day by day, and when this puberty thing is done she'll be an adult. Let's get beyond our resistance to her quest for independence, accept that it is her duty to need us less than she used to, and adjust to our new role as a parent of a budding teenager. And we can make our job and our child's transition to adolescence a lot easier by concentrating on what our child needs now as opposed to trying to keep her the child she was. Let's concentrate on how we become approachable during our child's pubertal and adolescent years.

You can start with your eight-year-old while he's still the child that you've always known him to be. Beginning our talks on puberty and sexual intercourse at this age allows us to establish ourselves as an approachable parent *before* the moon becomes full and our little boy begins to change into something else. By the time he does become that something else you will already have had several years of important conversations and discussions with him about some critical aspects of puberty and sexual behavior. If you do this correctly you will win out over his peers, the media, and any other significant influence on his sexual behavior and sexuality.

Here are some basic pointers to get you started. Again, try to become comfortable. If you already are, then great—you are one step ahead. You don't have to be "cool," and you don't have to try to impress your kid— you don't want to sound like one of his buddies. Remember, you are a parent, not a friend; you want him to view you as Mom or Dad who just happens to be able to talk to him about sex stuff. Again, you can start with the easy stuff, or you can dive right into the deep end.

Other parents have found the basic approach offered here to be a natural and effective starting point; we'll start with your daughter and then present a variation for your son.

I also believe that boys need to understand the changes that girls will go through, and girls need to understand all the ones that boys will experience. But this is more important for ten-, eleven-, and twelve-year-olds. For your eight-year-old you will keep your discussion gender specific; again, you only need to touch upon the basic changes of puberty.

A "Basics" Talk with Your Eight-Year-Old Daughter

"You know, I can't believe how big you're getting."

"I sure am," your daughter says proudly.

"I wonder when you're going to start puberty." She may already know what you're talking about, or think she does. But you want her to hear it from you. "That's when your body changes and you start turning into an adult. Do you want me to tell you what happens?"

If she seems hesitant, reassure her that this is something that happens to everyone—that it even happened to you—and then maybe name some other adults or older peers she likes and respects.

"There's no particular age that someone starts puberty. It could be at ten, eleven, or twelve; it could be earlier at nine or even later, like thirteen. What's important to know is that when it starts, that's the right time for you. And there are going to be a whole bunch of changes. It's all because of chemicals in your body called hormones. Your body starts to make a lot of these hormones, and bingo: you start to have puberty changes.

"Your breasts will grow, your shape will change, and your hips will widen a bit. You'll get your period, your ovaries will start to make one mature or grown-up egg cell a month, and you'll grow hair around your vagina and under your arms. You'll probably even get some pimples."

That's a lot for her to take in, so say something comforting now. "It's hard to say in what order these changes will occur, because everyone's different. But you know you can always come to me with any questions you might have."

"Yeah, okay, whatever you say." She looks relieved that the conversation is over.

In addition, I encourage you to highlight the following information for your daughter.

Menstruation. You may want to revisit my earlier description of menstruation (see page 136). You want your daughter to appreciate how amazing the whole biological process of preparing for possible pregnancy is. That is why your daughter will get her period—because her body now produces a mature ovum (egg cell) every month and at the same time it must prepare the uterus to receive that ovum should a sperm cell fertilize it. Think about that—a woman's body prepares itself every month for a possible pregnancy. Her uterine lining becomes engorged with extra blood just before she makes a mature ovum. After it implants itself in the uterus, in its very early stages of development the fertilized ovum will receive its nutrition from that blood-engorged lining of the uterus. If the woman's ovum is not fertilized the uterus will shed its extra blood and she will have her period. You will want to make sure that your daughter understands that she ovulates about twelve to fourteen days prior to her first day of menstruation each month: "When you start to menstruate it means that your body is now producing a mature egg cell called an ovum every month. Your body is now capable of becoming pregnant. Even though you are way too young to even think about becoming pregnant, your body is capable of pregnancy once you start to ovulate (make a mature ovum). And you will know when you have begun to ovulate when you get your period for the first time. We will have many discussions about not having sex until you are an adult, and about how to avoid getting pregnant when you don't want to."

Body image. This is such a *big* issue throughout the adolescent years. Your daughter will need to hear from you that she is lovable and capable inside and out. Help her to understand the limitations of physical attractiveness. Help her to see that the core values of a person, along with the good deeds the person has done, mean far more than any reflection in a mirror. She needs to learn to be herself and not to try to become what someone else is.

Make sense of sexual feelings. Your daughter has no doubt experienced some sexual feelings, most likely from masturbation. She may have some thoughts about another child being cute or appealing, but she likely has very few reference points for understanding sexual feelings for another person. I suggest you start a conversation with her about these feelings in a matter-of-fact manner. Here's a possible script:

"One of the changes you're going to go through during puberty is that you will begin to develop sexual feelings for other people. I know you're still several years away from having those feelings, but they will come. There'll be that certain someone who will kind of make your heart flutter and give you a butterflies-in-the-stomach feeling. I know it may seem a little weird but these feelings will be part of what will make you want to have sex one day with another person. You know how you like to masturbate sometimes? The feelings you have from that are similar to the feelings you'll actually have for another person. There are many people, teenagers and adults, who have allowed their sexual feelings to get the best of them. That is, they have sex when they really weren't ready for it or really shouldn't have done it. That's a major reason why so many teenagers get pregnant in this country every year. These kids were not able to control their sexual feelings."

Lay this foundation now, and it will be easier to continue similar discussions by the time she's ten—and even easier when you are getting into some very nitty-gritty talks at ages twelve and thirteen.

BEAUTY *IS* ONLY SKIN DEEP

One way I help kids better understand the limits of physical attractiveness is to highlight for them how we perceive people's physical looks after we have gotten to know them personally. It never fails that should we view a person as nice their physical attractiveness improves. If we view a person as a jerk their physical attractiveness lessens. The reason for this is that we come to see that the soul of a person, not his or her physical aspects, really does define who that person is.

A "Basics" Talk with Your Eight-Year-Old Son

With a son, these are the changes to cover:

"Your penis and testicles will grow larger, and your testicles will start to make sperm and semen. Your voice will change and your penis will change! That's right; it'll start to grow larger and will probably get stiff and hard a lot for no reason at all. In fact, I bet your penis even gets stiff and hard now; it's totally natural you know, even if it happens for no sexy reason at all. But during puberty it'll happen a whole lot."

Your son may be amazed at this point. He gets erections often, but he'll be stunned that you're calling him out on it. He'll think you are a genius for sure; he thought no one knew! Your son needs to have discussions with you around sexual feelings, body image, and the notion that puberty occurs for each individual when it is the right time for that person.

In addition, your eight-year-old son also must hear about the following:

Erections. Have a talk with your son about getting erections regularly; refer back to what I said about this earlier in the chapter. Tell him that if it ever happens in public he should remain cool and calm and it will go back to normal.

Wet dreams. Give him some insight into the fact that one day he'll likely have a wet dream. Explain to him that his testicles are making sperm and his body is making semen, and that at any time during puberty he could experience a wet dream. It's no big deal and it could well happen more than once.

Shrinkage: it's normal. I think it's important to mention the fact that the testicles and penis can really shrivel up, temporarily. The first time it happened to me I thought my testicles wouldn't come back down. I realized on my own that my fears were unfounded. But this is one of those things that can cause a young boy some real concern, so help him through this.

What Your Nine- and Ten-Year-Old Needs to Know

Simply stated, you want your ten-year-old to know everything that you would want any child going through puberty to know. Something happens when your kid gets into fifth grade. She is now part of the "senior graduating class" of an elementary school and there is a built-in sort of belief that she is now on the threshold of being a young woman. The same can be said of the boys as they are now about to go on and become young men. You can see budding boy-girl relationships starting to take hold, group-dates actually start popping up, and no doubt similar awakenings for the gay and lesbian kids (except they realize there's no public outlet in which to express their nascent sexuality).

So much developmental change occurs from September to June of fifth grade; just ask any fifth-grade teacher. Students come in the first day of school pretty much kid-like and leave as little grown-ups. "It's the hormones, Dr. Fred," so many teachers say to me. "They are far more aware in the spring than when they first came into my class." It is abundantly clear that many ten-year-olds start to develop newfound sexual feelings. The girls for the most part start to develop them earlier than the boys do, but there are plenty of boys who do as well.

Having said all this, let's get to the really important things that you should discuss with your nine- and ten-year-old about puberty. You will want to cover as well all the points I stated earlier, but these are the really important ones. I am not separating out the issues specific to either gender. They can now hear changes that are relevant to both genders. You can make the decision about how much you want to focus on the other gender's changes, but you should certainly go over them with your child.

Body image. Your ten-year-old has likely started some pubertal changes, particularly if she is in the later stages of her tenth year. As her body changes you want to keep her on an even keel with regard to how she perceives herself. So you need to keep coming back to talking points that tell her she is normal; she needs to eat well and exercise regularly; she should be proud of her uniqueness; physical beauty is truly only skin deep; and it's one's values and soul that defines a person. Explain to your child why she is lovable and capable, and highlight for her the things she does well. When you compliment your child make sure you explain why you are complimenting her. The goal here is to keep your child as comfortable in her skin as is possible.

Personal hygiene. Work with your child on establishing good habits. Important points to cover are the increase in sweating; bacteria growth on the skin; washing every part of the body every day; washing under one's foreskin of the penis if uncircumcised; and the connection between facial oil, bacteria, shedding of skin cells, and pimples.

Sexual feelings. Your conversations about understanding and managing them will become more frequent over time. You won't talk them to death but you will over the next several years want to impress upon your child the major responsibility one has to behave sexually in a healthy and risk-free way. One primary way your child will do that is by moderating his sexual feelings.

Reproduction basics. Elaborate more on the reproductive parts of the body and what happens when a sperm cell meets an egg cell. I've found that ten-year-olds love to hear about the whole process. Encourage looking at a book that depicts the internal reproductive parts of a woman and man. Both boys and girls need to be able to visualize how various organs are configured. You can explain the following:

- An egg cell lives for only twenty-four hours after being released from an ovary.
- Sperm cells can live inside a woman's uterus and fallopian tubes for several days.
- An egg cell is almost always fertilized in the fallopian tube.
- When a sperm cell enters an egg cell, the egg cell creates a protective barrier keeping other sperm cells out.
- When the sperm cell joins with the egg cell, the body of the sperm goes into the egg cell and its tail falls off.

You can compare and contrast these facts:

- A man's testicles are basically the same size as a woman's ovaries.
- A man's testicles make tens of millions of sperm a day, whereas an ovary makes one mature ovum a month.

- A man's testicles will make sperm up until the day he dies, whereas a woman's body will stop making mature egg cells around mid-life.

- Both men and women have breasts; a woman's are just bigger.

- A uterus can expand greatly to hold a developing baby.

- A vagina lengthens and widens when a woman becomes sexually excited, very much like a man's penis does.

I hope you can see that covering pubertal changes and reproductive facts is really rather easy. The harder part comes next: discussing and having conversations about sexual relationships, sexual intercourse, and how to actually manage sexual feelings. I will take you through some of the different scripts you can use, along with some examples of authentic instruction.

Age Eight: Introducing a More Detailed Discussion of Sexual Intercourse

What I have to say here is relevant for kids ages eight through ten. I think the concept of sexual intercourse is something that an eight-year-old can handle not only from a cognitive and intellectual standpoint but also from an affective or emotional point of view. For the most part, eight-year-olds still think sex is kind of yucky. They're getting there but they still are mostly removed from having any interest in sex. "Oh, Dad (or Mom), that's gross and disgusting" is a comment that you'll probably hear when you broach the subject. But do not be dismayed; you are continuing to open the door to being a wonderful, approachable parent, and a discussion of sexual intercourse now will lay a strong foundation for the additional information you offer when your child turns nine and ten and beyond.

At eight, children are in third grade and kind of considered part of the upper grades. Their social thinking is starting to develop and as a result some things that are sexual are beginning to pique their interest. But it is still very likely they will think all of it is yucky, or at least pretty weird. Nevertheless, they are capable of digesting the basics of what sexual intercourse is, why people have sexual intercourse, when and under what conditions people should have intercourse, and with whom they should have intercourse. They just don't want to be overwhelmed with your talk. They are, after all, some time away from actually having to think about having sex.

So what exactly should you say, and when should you say it? Over the next few pages, you'll read the way I normally answer those questions for parents. You don't have to treat my words as a script, of course. You can go in a different order or choose different scenarios. These are just suggestions to help you get the conversations going. Good luck!

That First Conversation

There is no particular time or place that you need to consider when initiating your discussion about sexual intercourse. Do establish a level of privacy; don't attempt it in front of anyone else, except your partner. And don't attempt it when your kid has a gaming device in his hand or is watching a movie and could become easily distracted.

Don't worry too much about how you're going to sound; just be yourself. The key is to get the conversation going; once that happens everything will fall into place. As for the actual words, you can try some variation of this:

"I want to have a really important discussion with you. I hope you know you can talk about anything with me, and that includes sexual stuff. I want to talk to you about sexual intercourse because I love you, and I want to make sure that you get this information from me or your dad (or mom)."

Make sure you're looking your child squarely in the eyes. Lean in to let him or her know you want to connect, and ensure that your body language signals comfort and reassurance. "Do you remember when I told you that to make a baby the man's sperm cell and the woman's egg cell must join together?" Feel free to draw a picture if it helps, and then continue.

"Well, have you ever wondered how those cells get together? It's like this: The sperm cell gets into the woman's body when the man puts his penis into the woman's vagina. It's called sexual intercourse. The man's penis becomes stiff or erect and he is able to then put it into the woman's vagina. And while the penis is in there, sperm cells and a fluid called semen come out of it and the sperm move like crazy toward the egg. It's a race for them, because whichever cell gets there first is the one that makes the baby." Turning it into a fun competition at the cellular level may take away some of the discomfort of what you've just described, without glossing over it.

Finally, explain that a woman's body makes one egg cell a month, and, if she has sexual intercourse when the egg cell is released, that's when she's most likely to get pregnant.

There, you've done it! It wasn't any harder than explaining the rules of a game. How do you think you did? You may still have a lot of smoothing out to do, but the part you were most worried about is done. Sure, your kid is probably rolling her eyes right about now, or maybe even making some noises indicating her discomfort, but you have just had your first "doing it" talk and nobody burst into flames. This is the first of many, but the first is always the toughest. So take a second to congratulate yourself.

Pay Attention to Your Child's Response

Notice how your child is doing. Chances are you can keep things going right now. But if she is feeling too uncomfortable, then you can tell her it's okay to stop for now. Be sure to share how much you care about her, and express how glad you are that you can talk like this. Then all you have to do is say you'll continue your discussion at another time. Invite your child to bring it up whenever she's ready.

With eight-year-olds, it's pretty hard to tell how they're connecting with some of these sex talks. You're discussing sexual intercourse, sexual feelings—things they have few reference points for, and reasonably have some difficulty relating to. This is very similar to you telling them about how drugs and cigarettes are bad for them; they're not there yet in their own lives, so they don't necessarily get it. But we all know now how important it is to get the drug and smoking message across early in their lives. Well, it's the same thing with sex. So don't waste any time worrying about whether you said everything exactly right—be glad that you've said it at all.

Sex as More Than Just Baby-Making

Whenever you do come back to discussing intercourse you will want to try to introduce the idea that people have sex for reasons other than just wanting to make a baby. That is, when people have sex they're basically doing it for enjoyment. Up to now you have discussed sexual intercourse within the context of procreation. But let's face it: at some point you need to tell your child that most people have sex because, well, it's a whole lot of fun to do. Eight years of age is not too young to find this out: "There are many adults who have sexual intercourse because they love the person they have sex with. Sex can feel good, it can make you feel closer to the person you love, it can provide incredible satisfaction, and it can make a couple's relationship better. The bottom line is sex can be fun."

Wow, telling your eight-year-old that adults have sex for reasons other than making a baby! Now, that's a big statement and a major step forward. But you have to keep your head and remember that you need to define the context in which intercourse should occur and the values that should be associated with it. This is of course just the beginning of many discussions about intercourse, as you will be lending plenty of guidance on many occasions throughout your child's teenage years. But you want to provide a foundation right from the get-go that confirms the conditions under which she or he should have sexual intercourse. So you might say, for example, "I firmly believe that you will have a happier life if you wait to have sex until you are an adult and you have found a person you love and who also loves you, someone you can fully trust, someone who respects you and whom you respect."

This message becomes increasingly important as your child becomes older, because there will be many competing messages and challenges to it. But the idea here is to start early and scaffold or build upon what you teach each time you have a discussion with your child. A child who is only eight is not really going to connect with your discussions of sex as well as he will when he is ten. But by starting now rather than later, you have laid the foundation.

Age eight is also a good time to introduce the idea that HIV can be transmitted through sexual intercourse: "You know how I have talked to you about HIV and AIDS; if a woman has HIV in her body she has lots of it in the wetness inside her vagina. If a man has HIV he has lots of it in his sperm cells and the fluid semen that the sperm cells are in. If a person with HIV has sexual intercourse with another person, HIV can be spread to that person."

Ages Nine and Ten: Beyond Intercourse

You can begin to discuss much more about sexual behavior when your child gets to nine and ten years of age. You will extend your discussions about sexual intercourse; the role of love, respect, and trust; and when and with whom to have sexual intercourse. You can also begin to talk about the use of a condom, oral and anal intercourse, peer pressure, some basic thoughts about dating, and of course sexual feelings. You will want to make sure to cover the points I made earlier on sexual relationship behavior. Your kid may still think some of this is "yucky" and "gross," but you'll likely encounter less of this resistance. As your child gets closer and closer to puberty he will become more and more interested in your discussions about sexual behavior. This is an important fact for you to remember. Your child will really want to hear more about puberty and sexual behavior when he's ten, eleven, and twelve years of age. If you solidify your role as an approachable mentor during these earlier years you will have it much easier as your child transitions to middle and high school.

What's It Really Like?

I have found that many nine-year-olds and certainly ten-year-olds have heard quite a bit about sexual intercourse, even if what they've learned hasn't come from their parents. They're still fairly naive about specifics, but for the most part they know that the penis goes into the vagina. Consequently, they are very inquisitive about exactly how it feels to have intercourse and the actual mechanics that go into it.

You can say to your child, "You know how we've discussed what sexual intercourse is, and how people who are in love have sex because it makes them feel closer and it feels good?"

"Yeah," your child says, very sure that you're going to have one of your sex talks.

"Well, have you ever wondered exactly what the man and woman do and how it actually feels?" you ask her.

"Ah, well, sort of," your daughter replies, knowing full well that she's still going to get a talking-to. (One of the really neat things about being a parent who is approachable on sexual matters is that you always get a familiar *here goes Mom [or Dad] again* response from your kid. He or she just comes to expect that this is a normal part of being with you, and it's one of many conversations you have.)

"It's important for both the man and woman to talk to each other about what feels good and what doesn't feel so great when they have sex. For example, the woman has to take her time a little at first, because her vagina actually has to widen and lengthen somewhat in order to be able to fit the penis inside her. If that hasn't happened when the man is ready, she needs to be able to tell him."

"You mean it wouldn't fit otherwise?" your daughter asks somewhat incredulously.

"Probably not, and it would certainly hurt somewhat. You see, the vagina also becomes wetter when the woman becomes excited and that takes a little time as well. So the vagina has to change size and become wetter in order for intercourse to be pleasurable."

"Okay," your daughter says. "What else would they have to talk about?"

"Well, when the penis is in her vagina the man moves his penis in and out and the woman sort of moves with him. Fast, slow, faster, slower, and sometimes it's pretty important to talk about what feels better in terms of the speed with which the penis moves in the vagina."

"I think I've heard enough, Mom, thanks." Your daughter gets up to go to her room.

"Okay, honey, it was nice having this little talk. You know how much I love you."

"Sure do, Mom. See ya." And up to her room she goes.

Can you see yourself having this conversation with your daughter or son? Kids this age really do have thoughts about what sex feels like.

I've had nine- and ten-year-olds ask me many times how sex feels and what the man and woman feel when they have sex. So now is the time to venture into those waters and be approachable on any question about sexual intercourse.

What About Abortion?

You will want to have some discussion with your nine- or ten-year-old child about abortion: "You know, now that I have discussed sexual intercourse with you, it is important that you understand what an abortion is. Abortion is the medical termination or end to a pregnancy. Unfortunately, there are women who become pregnant when they don't want to be. They have sexual intercourse but don't want to become pregnant. And, tragically, there are some women who are forced into sex and become pregnant. In the United States today, there are more than one million abortions that occur every year."[5] You will want to discuss your values and beliefs about abortion with your child, and I hope you will encourage her to feel secure in knowing that, irrespective of your beliefs and values, she could come to you should she ever find herself with an unintended pregnancy.

Whether you are talking to your daughter or son, the script is basically the same. You can continue by saying: "Sweetheart, I know I've spoken with you about not having sexual intercourse until you are an adult and in a loving, trusting, and respectful relationship. Yet, I need you to understand that I am always here for you. Should you or your partner ever have to face a pregnancy I am here for you. I don't think anyone ever wants to be faced with the decision of what to do if they or their partner has an unintended pregnancy. You need to learn how to be sexually responsible and avoid unintended pregnancy, and that is why we have our talks about sex."

Oral and Anal Sex

As you share your thoughts about sexual intercourse—the fact that you expect it to occur in adulthood, when in love, and with total respect and trust with the other person—you can then build in some discussion of different types of sexual intercourse: "Remember that we have talked about sexual intercourse. Well, sometimes adults who are in love will also put their mouth on the other person's private parts or genitals. The man will sometimes put his mouth on the woman's vulva and the woman will put her mouth on his penis. This is called oral sex or giving a blow job or giving head. Sometimes the man and woman will have anal intercourse. This is when the man puts his penis in the woman's rectum or rear end."

This little talk may bring a "yucky" or two but will be handled just fine by your child. I think most experts would agree that far too many teenagers are engaging in oral sex, not realizing the risks. Not only are there considerable numbers of teens who are engaging in both sexual intercourse and oral sex, but there are teens who have had oral sex as a way to avoid pregnancy or in the mistaken belief that this preserves their virginity. And while anal sex may not be as popular, this behavior nonetheless does occur among some teens and adolescents. I meet a lot of kids who truly believe that oral and anal sex are really not sex and many who think that oral sex is relatively harmless. Many of them believe that you're still a virgin if you have oral or anal sex. You certainly want to impress upon your nine- and ten-year-old that oral and anal sex are indeed sex:

"It's real important that you understand that there are a number of kids in middle and high school who are having oral sex. Some are even having anal sex. When you get into middle school you're going to hear about this and may even be asked or pressured by some people to do it."

Your son will look at you and say, "Don't worry, Dad, I'm never gonna do that."

"Yeah, well, one day you just might. Look, when you're an adult, having someone you love do that can feel really, really good. I'm not going to lie to you; I'll bet you'll want to have it done to you. And giving oral sex is also something that you'll probably want to do. I just want you to understand that all this stuff is out there and you're going to have to deal with it at some point. You know how much we've talked about waiting until you're an adult and in love to have sex. Well, that includes oral and anal sex."

By now your son has probably had enough and is ready to go back to whatever it is he has planned. He may well say, "Yeah, okay, can I go now?" He may well be somewhat embarrassed (and definitely will be if you haven't already been talking with him about sex). But all of this is ultimately for his benefit, so don't dismay.

At some point later you'll be able to pick up the conversation where you left off and make some mention of how anal or oral sex don't lead to pregnancy but are a way of transmitting HIV and other sexually transmitted infections: "I am so glad we talked the other day about oral and anal sex. I just wanted to say one other thing. Obviously, not having sexual intercourse or oral and anal sex is the best way to avoid getting HIV. But if someone decides to have sexual intercourse of any sort, the next best way to avoid getting HIV is for the man to wear a condom over his penis when he has sex. A condom is made of a material called latex. It comes rolled up in a package and when it is removed it can be rolled onto his penis before he has sexual intercourse or oral or anal sex."

If you have a daughter your conversations will be basically the same. It's a simple fact that for heterosexuals there is more girl-to-boy oral sex than there is boy-to-girl (although not a considerable difference), so keep this in mind.

Introducing your nine- and ten-year-old kids to these issues is an important step forward in preparing them for their journey into adolescence. So remember that what you're doing now gets this whole conversation going before your daughter or son has to confront anything having to do with oral or anal sex.

How Do Gays and Lesbians Do It?

I get this question often when having these discussions about sex with nine- and ten-year-olds. When I am asked, my answer is rather simple: "Well, they have sex pretty much like a man and a woman. They can have oral sex, and gay men can have anal sex if they choose. Some lesbian women, if they choose, can use a sex toy or dildo that they insert into their vaginas, which is very safe. A dildo is several inches long and kind of looks like a cucumber." When I say this in a matter-of-fact way, the kids usually aren't sure how they should react. Most seem rather amazed, others will giggle. I will usually end this talk by saying, "Remember, we must always respect anyone we think is different from us."

All About Condoms

One day, hopefully not until they become adults, most all of our kids will have sexual intercourse and possibly oral and anal intercourse as well. Irrespective of when they start to have sexual intercourse, they should absolutely use a condom. Even if they have absolute love, respect, and trust in their relationship and their partner is totally honest about not having any sort of sexually transmitted infection, and even if a form of contraception is already being used, it just makes sense to use a condom as an extra level of protection.

Discussing condoms and how to use them will *not* increase your child's likelihood of becoming sexually active. I suppose that if you just gave your kid a condom with no meaningful conversation, this could be seen as an invitation to give it a try. But that's not what you're going to do, right? If you share with your child your values about when and with whom to have sex and provide meaningful, authentic teaching about making good decisions, simply having a conversation with him about condoms isn't going to make him go out and try one. It will, however, improve his chances of never having to experience an unwanted pregnancy or sexually transmitted infection.

Yes, Your Kids Are Ready to Learn

My guess is your child will be riveted when you do explain to him how to use a condom. (Your daughter needs to learn this as well. I think she's too young to learn how to use a female condom, but she needs to be informed about how a male uses a condom.) Whenever I discuss how to use a condom with a group of nine- or ten-year-olds you can hear a pin drop.

Virtually every ten-year-old I have spoken to over the last several years seems to know what a condom is. They have heard that a condom is something a man wears on his penis that captures sperm so that it can't get a woman pregnant. Fewer of them know that a condom can help stop the spread of sexually transmitted infections and HIV, or that men who have sex with men might use them.

Condoms, Start to Finish

I've never liked using a banana or a cucumber to demonstrate how to put a condom on and take it off. I've always thought it makes light of a very important subject. I'm all for humor in the sex education classroom, but not when discussing what is such a serious issue as preventing a pregnancy or transmission of HIV. All you really need is a condom and your fingers to demonstrate. So get yourself a condom and let's show your nine- or ten-year-old how to use one:

"Before I show you how to use a condom I want you to understand that, just like crossing the street or playing tennis, using a condom correctly takes a certain amount of skill. A man or woman can't just wake up one day and know exactly how to use a condom. It takes some practice to develop the skills that are needed to use a condom correctly."

Your child will look at you like you've lost them a little.

"No, really. There are a number of things that a man needs to do right when using a condom or else it won't be as effective as it could be in preventing pregnancy or the spread of disease like the HIV virus. So I want you to pay special attention to what I say.

"First, all condoms have an expiration date on the box that they come in. They should not be used past that date. Condoms need to be stored at room temperature and kept out of sunlight or else they can go bad. For HIV protection, they must be made of latex or rubber. There is a variety now that is made of vinyl for people who are allergic to rubber or latex. Some condoms are made from lamb intestines, but only latex and vinyl condoms reduce the spread of HIV. When you open a condom's package, you will see that the condom is rolled up." Here you will open the condom package. "Make sure you tear the package at the end or else you could rip the condom.

"Before he can put it on, the man's penis must be erect and hard. First, the man must figure out which way the condom will be rolled out." Use your index and middle fingers to determine which way it will roll down. "If the man didn't do this first and just put the condom up against his penis and started rolling, what would happen if he tried rolling it down the wrong way?"

Using your fingers, show your child that the condom will roll down the penis only one way. Then explain:

"When a man is really sexually excited his penis can leak sperm and semen. This happens before he ejaculates. If the man tried rolling the condom down his penis the wrong way and the tip of the condom touches any sperm or semen that might be leaking from the man's penis, than there would now be some sperm and semen on the outside of the condom. So if the man turned it around and started rolling it down his penis, the sperm and semen on the outside of the condom could go into his partner's vagina, rectum, or mouth when he has intercourse.

"The man rolls the condom all the way down over the penis, this way." Now roll the condom down over your middle and index fingers.

"Now I want you to remember something that may not seem to have too much to do with how to use a condom, but it is very important. That is, when a couple has sex they should keep a light on. Sexual intercourse should happen with the light on! This is because sometimes a condom can rip or actually slide off the man's penis. And chances are good that he'd never realize it. That's because it feels virtually the same to have intercourse using a condom as it does when not using a condom. So the only way the man will know if the condom has torn or slipped off is to look periodically at his penis when having sex.

"After the man ejaculates he needs to hold the condom at its base against his penis as he takes his penis out of his partner's vagina or rectum." Show how you would hold the base of the condom. "The man does this so no semen spills into his partner's body. He then should wrap the used condom in tissue paper and throw it into the garbage."

Your nine- or ten-year-old will likely be amazed at all of this. Of course, you should remind your child about waiting until adulthood to have sex, and the whole love, respect, and trust thing should be mentioned. You should reassure her that you discuss these things because you want her to come to you first with any questions or concerns about sex, and you realize just how important this information for her is as she becomes an adolescent.

Anyone's Child Could Be Gay or Lesbian

I have discussed some issues that pertain to gays and lesbians already, as I think it's pretty important to teach your child to have an awareness of homosexuality, as well as to develop tolerance and acceptance for people who are gay or lesbian.

Every parent needs to be open to the possibility that their child is homosexual. Children pick up on the prevailing cultural message that heterosexuality is the norm and homosexuality is not. They also pick up on the many negative attitudes that exist toward homosexuality. So it's understandably common for gay kids to try to conceal their true sexual orientation. I think that if you work hard at being approachable on all matters sexual, then your child will be comfortable enough at some point to share with you whether or not he or she is gay. You both should understand that as your child enters puberty and travels through adolescence it will become increasingly clear to her whether she is heterosexual or homosexual.

Some parents feel compelled to ask their kids at some point whether they are straight or gay. I personally don't think it's such a big deal that you would have to ask. If you are open and approachable, then it is likely she'll tell you at some point. If you think or sense that she is a lesbian and you want to know, of course you can ask her if you want to. I recommend waiting until she's in high school. However, try to find opportunities well before then to recount a true story or two about a young gay or lesbian person who struggled with discrimination and how important it would have been for the young person to have gone to her parents for help. There are more than enough true stories about gay and lesbian teens and young adults who have gone through hell because of their sexual orientation. Discussing a story or two with your nine- or ten-year-old and then sharing your perspective as a parent is well advised.

When recounting the story, you could say something like, "I can tell you that if I were her parent I would totally accept and love her whether she was straight, homosexual, or bisexual. I would make sure that my gay son or lesbian daughter would feel safe and secure at all times. This is why I want you to feel totally comfortable coming to me with any, and I mean any, issue concerning sex or anything else that you might be dealing with. Because I love you and will always love you no matter what you do."

You can also weave in a story or two about young people who are transgender or young people who display their sexuality in ways that are contrary to society's norms, and the difficulty they have had growing up. (Transgender kids' gender identity—that is, their view of who they are as male, female, both, or something else—does not match their biological gender that they were born with and in no way is indicative of their particular sexual orientation.) Children whose sexuality doesn't fit societal norms can be quite varied. The important issue here for our kids is that anyone can express their sexuality in ways they see fit as long as it in no way negatively impacts others.

Seize the Day

Take advantage of teachable moments. They're more spontaneous, and they often help our children understand things better than one of those formal sit-down talks might, because they happen during the normal course of life.

A Teachable Moment: The TV Show

One way to start a conversation about sexual intercourse, or, for that matter, any other aspect of sexuality, is to use the media as a springboard. Here's an example: You are watching TV with your eight-year-old and there is a scene where two people meet each other at a bar, have a few drinks, and seem to enjoy each other's company. Later, as they are getting ready to leave, they decide to go to the woman's apartment for coffee. Arriving at the apartment, the two engage in friendly talk, the man slides his arm over her shoulder at some point, he leans in and kisses her, they fall back on the couch and start to pull off each other's clothes . . . and then the camera pans away and the scene fades to commercial.

You turn to your daughter with an incredulous look and say, "Did you just see what I just saw?"

"Yeah," she answers, looking up at you.

"Well, what do you think?"

"I don't know."

"Well, I think they're gonna have sex; I mean, they don't even know each other and they are getting naked and I think they're gonna have sex."

"That's really gross, Dad!"

"Yeah, but what do you really think about it? Do you think two people who just met each other should ever have sex? Really, tell me what you think."

"I don't think two people should ever have sex, Dad."

From her lips to God's ears, you think. *My daughter will never have sex.* You then jolt yourself back to reality.

"Well, let me tell you what I think," you soldier on. "They're nuts! They don't know anything about each other, one of them could have HIV or some other disease, and the other could get it. It's just like how we tell you not to get into a stranger's car!"

She remains silent, but you can tell she is mulling it over in her mind. "Do you know what other bad things could happen if they don't know anything about each other?"

"Um, no." She isn't entirely comfortable, but she isn't shutting you down, either.

"The guy could decide to force her or hurt her," you continue, still maintaining eye contact. "She could become pregnant. Or maybe one of them will decide to never see the other again—which would leave that other person feeling really used."

"What does *feeling used* mean?"

Aha! Questions are good! You should always remind yourself to pause often and wait for one—but keep in mind that just because they *don't* ask doesn't mean they don't still need to know.

"Well," you answer, "it's when you share something special with someone, and they don't appreciate it. If you feel like you're doing something special, the other person should, too."

You can see that your daughter is ready to move on from this conversation—she has not only stopped looking you in the eye, but also seems to be looking for a giant "exit" sign to run toward. So you acknowledge that it is okay for her to feel uncomfortable, and wrap it up.

"I can see that's enough for you," you say as you smile and nudge her gently. "But I'm so glad we had this talk, sweetheart. I know it's not easy to hear Dad talk like this, but having sex will be one of the biggest decisions you'll ever make in life. I want you to know you can come to me or Mom and have a private talk anytime."

The above example encourages the child to be able to come to mom as well as dad with any concerns. It's important to highlight here that if you don't have a partner, identify for your child a trusted adult of the other gender that she can always speak with, perhaps a relative or trusted friend. I recommend this even if you're a gay or lesbian couple, because hearing from another gender can be important for your child, just for a different perspective.

A Teachable Moment: At the Neighbor's

Teachable moments can happen anywhere, anytime. Say you've just stopped by your neighbor's home with your eight-year-old son and she is in the middle of an argument with her teenage son after finding him alone with his girlfriend in his bedroom. Now, the polite thing to do would be to cover your kid's ears, silently slip out the door, and pretend not to have heard anything. And you can still do that! But remember that this is also an opportunity to share your thoughts and values with your child. All parents will confront this issue at some point: at what age do you allow your adolescent to have private time with his or her "friend" in your home? This is a perfect opportunity for discussion: there's no time like the present to start laying some groundwork on this particular issue.

Once you have some privacy with your child, you can have the conversation go something like this:

"I want to talk with you a little bit about what happened over at the neighbor's house. She was upset with her son because he had been alone in his bedroom with his girlfriend. Do you know why that might upset his mom?"

Start off by discussing that and then take it a bit further. "I don't think they were having sex, but I do think that his mom was afraid that they might."

You've set up why there was tension in the other house, now it's time to communicate how you would feel in a similar situation. "I would also be upset if he was my son, or if it were you at sixteen. I just think a kid that age is too young to be alone with his girlfriend in his bedroom."

Now tell him why. "My guess is he has probably developed some pretty strong sexual feelings and as a parent I always worry about teenagers being able to control them. You will learn more about sexual feelings when you get older. And you'll develop them as you go through puberty. Everyone has to learn how to control his or her sexual feelings—and it's not easy."

Teachable moments are a wonderful way to explore issues of sex and sexuality that your child soon may face. When we don't take advantage of teachable moments we miss golden opportunities to reinforce what we as parents believe to be important information or messages that our kids need to learn. So, for example, if your child is listening to a particular song whose lyrics are disrespectful and denigrating to women, and you don't ask what the child thinks about the lyrics, or how it makes him feel when he hears someone sing about women like that, or whether he thinks that other kids hearing those lyrics think that that's how girls and women should be treated, then you are missing a great opportunity to help your child reflect on how misguided and demeaning messages about women can be hurtful and dangerous.

Teachable moments can represent both positive and negative messages about sex and sexuality. The positive messages, like a teacher intervening when she sees a form of sexual harassment occurring, or a character in a TV show who refuses to have sex when pressured to do so, can be reinforced with your child by using a few simple reflective questions: "Do you agree with what the teacher did or what the TV character did? Why or why not? If the teacher hadn't intervened, what else might have happened? How do you think the student being harassed felt? If the TV character had not stood up to the peer pressure she was experiencing, what could happen if she did have sex?" Likewise, if the teachable moment message is negative, like the lyrics in the above example, you will strengthen your child immeasurably by helping him see the destructiveness of such lyrics. Having him explore what it means to celebrate a music artist who makes money and gains fame by singing at the expense of women will help him to develop a responsible insight into the impact the media have on culture and society.

Sexual Feelings

As I've said all along, the biggest change of puberty your child will likely grapple with is the development of sexual feelings. Your nine- or ten-year-old is not quite there yet, but now is the perfect time to introduce them to your kids.

Tell your child that if he was in second grade and you asked him what he thought of the girls he'd probably say something like, "Ah, who needs them?" And if there was a fourth- or fifth-grade girl in the room and she was asked what she thought of the boys back in second grade, she too would probably say something similar. But if you were to ask him and perhaps some other fifth- and fourth-grade boys and girls what they think of the opposite sex now, some would say, "Hmm, they're really not so bad after all." In fact, some would say that some of those boys or girls are cute or pretty or sexy. There are even some boys who would think other boys are cute and some girls who would think some of the other girls are pretty. You can say, "That is because some kids your age are starting to develop sexual feelings. Many will have heterosexual feelings and some will have homosexual feelings. When you get into middle school these sexual feelings will become stronger and then even more so when you get into high school.

"So let's pretend for a moment that you are fifteen years old and in tenth grade. What would you say and do if a really gorgeous guy or girl whom you think is nice came onto you? Wanted to kiss you? Or, suppose you actually know this person and you're pretty sure that he or she has looked at you on a number of occasions, and in fact, you think he or she actually likes you. What would you do?"

My guess is your nine- or ten-year-old will not be keen on the idea of kissing; some will, but most will say, "I wouldn't kiss her or him."

But irrespective of what your child tells you, you continue, "Now remember, you're pretending to be fifteen, so after wanting to kiss you he or she then touches your leg and tries to touch your penis or vagina. What would you say and do?"

Again, I would bet that your child would say, "Nope, not me. I would say, 'get your hands off me,' and then I would leave."

Your job at this point is to highlight for your child that his sexual feelings would be pretty strong at fifteen, much stronger than they are now, and likely would be compelling him to allow the touches to happen:

"I don't know about that. Your sexual feelings might be really strong at fifteen. Remember, you like this person and they are showing you a lot of affection and I bet it would be tough not to give in. If you could speak to yourself in the future what would you say to yourself about being in this position?"

AUTHENTIC INSTRUCTION SUGGESTIONS

1. Role-play with your child some situations where his sexual feelings are being challenged; have him act out how he would handle the situation. For example, your child is at a party in middle school and someone suggests they leave to go somewhere more private with a bunch of other kids who want to "hook up" with them. A girl says to him, "I can't wait to be alone with you."

2. Practice letter writing: Have your child pretend *she* is a parent and write a letter to her daughter or son explaining how she should manage her sexual feelings when they emerge. In the voice of a parent, your child would describe how she would want "her child" to handle her sexual feelings, what values are needed in order to manage her feelings, and the potential impact on herself and others if she were to act on her sexual feelings or not.

3. Do a cost-benefit analysis of a situation in which a fourteen-year-old allows his sexual feelings to get the best of him and engages in sexual intercourse. Have your child identify and discuss the benefits and the risks of engaging in sexual intercourse.

You want your child to actually give advice to herself in this future scenario. You want her to talk about being strong and not giving in to her sexual feelings. To talk about how she would say no; what she would do if he didn't want to stop kissing or touching her; what she could have done right after the first kiss and before he touched her. You want her to think of actions she can take to avoid any unwanted sexual contact even though there may be a part of her (her sexual feelings) that enjoys the kissing and the touching.

The key to having authentic discussions with your child around sexual feelings is to focus on things your child can actually do when faced with those feelings. In this example you focused on what your child would say to her future self about a particular life situation she could one day find herself in. See the sidebar for some other possibilities for authentic instruction.

Peer Pressure

I mentioned earlier the incredible influence that peers can have on our children as they grow and develop into adolescents. It is crucial that as parents we establish ourselves as approachable before our kids hit middle school, because peer group influence will take on a higher level of significance than our kids have had to confront. Just as we did with sexual feelings, we have an obligation to use authentic strategies to help our kids deal with peer pressure situations.

Create for your child a situation where she is already in middle school and some of her peers have been approaching her lately trying to befriend her. One of the leaders of the group comes up to her one day and invites her to a party. She says that she and her other friends decided to invite her because they think she'd be fun to hang with. The leader says there are going to be boys at the party, and some beer and other alcohol, and the best part is that the parents of the kid hosting the party won't be home. "You do want to come, don't you?" asks the leader.

Stop there and ask your child what she would do. Remember, you want your nine or ten-year-old to reflect on the consequences of the decision she will make. Should she go or shouldn't she? If she says no, what will the leader and the others in the group say or do? What if they make fun of her when she says no; how will she handle that? If she goes to the party, what are the possible consequences? These are the sorts of questions that will help your child understand what can happen if she does or doesn't stand up to negative peer pressure.

AUTHENTIC TEACHING STRATEGIES FOR PEER PRESSURE

1. Do a role-play exercise with your child about being pressured to do something that he's not sure he should be doing.

2. Introduce to your child the concept of the "uh-oh" feeling that we get when we are confronted with something that just doesn't feel right. Think of a variety of situations that you could pose to your child that might or might not create an "uh-oh" feeling and have him tell you which ones might cause this feeling and which would not. Have your child explain why he would or wouldn't have that feeling in each situation and talk together about whether or not you think his feelings were on target. Situations could include the following:

   - Being asked to keep a birthday secret from his mother
   - Being asked to keep secret from his parents that he was asked to drink beer at a peer's house
   - Being asked to give oral sex to a girl at a party
   - Being asked to participate in a prank where boys drop a book in front of a girl and then try to look up her skirt when she bends over to pick it up

Sexual Decision Making

The same strategies you teach your child to use in understanding sexual feelings and dealing with peer pressure can be used for sexual decision making. Having your child practice making decisions in hypothetical sexual situations will help her when she is confronted with similar situations in real life. When I speak to kids in the fourth and fifth grades I always remind them that some of the biggest decisions they will ever make in life concern sex and sexuality. Making the wrong decision could mean the difference between life and death or happiness and despair. You need to convey this sense of urgency to your child. Here are some possible strategies:

1. Make up as many scenarios that would require sexual decision making as you can. A scenario should include a major decision that your child may have to make in real life during adolescence. In addition to the situations mentioned under managing sexual feelings and peer pressure, try these:

   • What would you do if a really beautiful and very popular guy or girl wanted to have sex with you but that person is known to have sex with people and then leave them? What would you say and do? How do you think you would feel after making your decision? Describe what you think your parents and your friends would say about your decision.

   • Suppose you're dating someone in high school and that person says he/she really loves you and wants to have sex with you. You feel that you love her or him as well. Would you go ahead and have sex? Why, or why not? What if you didn't want to but your boyfriend or girlfriend did? Describe what you think would happen if you went ahead and had sex. What would happen if you decided not to?

- Suppose you're in eighth grade and all your good friends are telling you to go ahead and have sex with a guy or girl you really, really like. How would you handle that? Think of as many different ways of handling that situation as you can. Map out the consequences for each way of handling it.

- Imagine you are in middle school and you're at a party at the house of one of your classmates. A bunch of boys and girls are there and you're enjoying yourself. A friend of yours asks you to come into another room and when you enter you see some girls giving blow jobs to two boys. Your friend wants you to join her in giving oral sex to the boys as well. What would be your reaction? How would you deal with this? What would you say or do? What would you think of your friend?

2. The scenarios don't have to deal only with making decisions about having sex. What about dating? Here are some possibilities:

- Suppose you are in middle school, in sixth grade, and you're asked out on a date. If you thought the guy or girl was nice, would you go? Why, or why not? What do you think your parents would say? What is the right time to begin dating? What are the advantages of group dating as opposed to one-on-one dating? What would happen if you went out with a group of boys and girls in seventh grade and a few of the kids wanted to change plans and go somewhere different from where you had told your parents you were going to go? What would your choices be, and how would you go about implementing the one you would choose?

- Suppose several of your fellow fourth-grade students started making fun of your breasts, which are starting to develop. How would you handle that? What would you say or do? Would you tell anyone? Whom would you tell? Or, suppose several of your classmates wanted you to join with them to tell one of the boys that he has a really good-looking butt? What would you say or do? Why? Would you tell anyone? Whom would you tell? Or, suppose several of your classmates wanted you to join in making fun of a fellow student's breasts. What would you say or do? Why? Would you tell anyone? Whom would you tell?

We've waded into some pretty interesting territory here. Again, it's all about being an approachable parent. Practicing these decisions in hypothetical situations like this will arm your child to resist some of the nasty and bad things that can come from irresponsible sexual decision making.

QUESTIONS FROM TEN-YEAR-OLDS

To give you some insight into what your ten-year-old may ask about sex and sexuality, I have listed below some of the actual questions ten-year-olds have written anonymously on an index card prior to my visit to their classroom. (An "m" or an "f" indicates whether the question was asked by a male or female student.)

1. At what age should you start having sex? (f)

2. What is the proper age to have sex? (m)

3. Do you have to die after sex if you have sex with someone who has AIDS? (m)

4. How do people have sex? (m)

5. How do you get a girlfriend? (m)

6. Is it true you get herpes around the mouth area? (f)

7. What is rimming? (m)

8. How long do you have to do sex to have a baby? (f)

9. If you have sex and you push very hard will a man or woman have an asthma attack? (f)

10. Why do daddies suck our mothers' breasts? (m)

11. If a girl has sex and she doesn't have safe sex, does it means she gets pregnant? (f)

12. Why are abortions legal? (f)

13. How does it feel to have sex? Hard? Good? Bad? Half/half? (m)

14. Do you really bleed the first time you have sex? (f)

15. What happens when you have sex and what goes on in your body? (m)

16. If you wear a condom can you still get pregnant? If so, how does it get through? (f)

17. What percent of STDs can be cured? (m)

18. What do you do if someone tries to rape you? (m)

19. What's an orgasm? (m)

20. How do you prevent peer pressure toward sex? (f)

21. How come men need a boner to have sex? (m)

22. Is it really terrible to have sex before you're married? (f)

23. What about sex do you have to be careful about? (f)

24. Should sex be pleasurable? (f)

25. Why do people jerk off? (m)

Keep in mind, the kids asked these questions *before* I came to their class and before they had any sex education at their school. How do you think you would do in answering these questions? We've discussed the answers to most of them already somewhere within this book. Also, keep in mind that it is important that you don't wait for your kids to come to you. Some kids will never come to you with questions, so it's up to you to get the conversation started and keep it going.

Final Thoughts on Preparing for Puberty

You will want to have had significant conversations about sex and sexuality with your child before he or she enters middle school. If you wait until then to initiate talks about when and with whom to have sex, it will likely be more difficult to influence your child than it would have been if you had started much earlier. Eight, nine, and ten are the perfect ages to begin very important talks about sexual intercourse. This is because it is always much easier to reinforce the concept of abstinence at a time when your young child has no desire to be sexually active. At ten years of age the prevailing desire and expectation among your child and his peer group is to remain chaste until adulthood—if not until death! When we make a sincere effort to reinforce this belief while they themselves still believe it, we have a better chance that our children will remain abstinent the remainder of their adolescent years.

CHAPTER 9

Middle School and Beyond

Let's look at the middle school years now. Whether you've just picked up this book and are playing catch-up, or you have already laid the foundation for your being approachable and your child's number one source of sex information, sex has most likely been theoretical for your child before middle school. Starting with middle school, however, you face an unavoidable question: How much sexual behavior should adolescents engage in?

I've offered my opinion that a little "fooling around" by your adolescent is not all bad. Now that you are planning for the middle and high school years, it's important to identify exactly what is acceptable sexual behavior for your budding adolescent. It is important to consider the role of adolescence in helping us learn about our eventual sexual roles as adults. Think about your own adolescence: the sexual experiences you had then helped to refine and define to some degree your sexual experiences in early adulthood. In other words, one stage of life helps to prepare us for the next stage, and so on. Whether good or bad, we all learn from our sexual experiences, and we hope that the bad experiences are minimal and involve nothing that is life threatening. Unfortunately, when it comes to sexual behavior, the bad can be very bad. That is why I have gone to the effort of helping you learn how to get your child through to adulthood with a minimum of harm.

To think that a young person should have no sexual experiences until adulthood is naive and probably not very healthy. There should be some "fooling around," some tryout experiences—as long as your teen is prepared to manage and control those experiences so that risk of harm is minimized to its lowest common denominator. So let's make a list of some of the sexually related behaviors that our teen might engage in and the conditions and circumstances in which they might occur, and discuss each in turn.

Kissing

I cannot imagine our children going through adolescence without kissing; can you? Most of us remember our first few kisses, and I don't know about you but some of the best times I had during my adolescence were the heavy-duty make-out sessions. Of course, the sexual feelings you can get from these sessions can at times be overwhelming and can certainly prime us to want to go further. But it's going a little too far to say our kids aren't allowed to kiss. And that goes for kids in middle school, not just high school. You may have some difficulty with the idea of your sixth or seventh grader kissing and making out, but I really can't see any problem with it as long as you have had your share of discussions about how he would need to manage his feelings and behavior. To be clear, I am certainly not suggesting that you encourage your child to engage in kissing sessions.

So now that we've decided that kissing is okay, how about tongue kissing? Well, I do stand on the side of tongue kissing, but I say that we need to choose carefully the person we want to do this with. I have had many discussions with middle school students about tongue kissing and I always ask them, "What if the person you're tongue kissing likes to eat her or his boogers?" They always respond, "Oh man, Dr. Fred, that's really gross!" but it does give them pause. On the serious side, when you address this with your children just make sure you discuss with them the possible urge to go further than just kissing.

Feeling Up and Feeling Down
Over the Clothes

When teens go beyond kissing, they generally try touching either the breasts or the genitals. You need to set boundaries and conditions: mainly, I suggest limiting your endorsement of this behavior to high school students only (but more on this shortly). You should only permit trying this behavior out with someone the teen trusts and respects. (True love may be too much to ask for at this stage, but teens should at least limit these experiences to someone with whom they feel real affection—not just lust.) Here's where all your prior talks about respect and trust will pay off. But we must realize that when teens start feeling up and down, the urge to go further is very real. The next step is to explore with your teen how she would expect to keep things under control and not go any further than just touching.

Again, I think our middle school kids are too young for this. What do you think? Do you want your eleven-, twelve-, or thirteen-year-old son or daughter feeling or getting felt up? I'm guessing most of you will agree with me. If you do, you will need to discuss with your middle school child how to avoid these behaviors.

Feeling Up and Down *Under* the Clothes

Now things are starting to get a little dicey, wouldn't you say? Touching the breasts or genitals under the clothes is going to make things very hot, perhaps much too hot for teenagers to handle.

This is where I would hope my teen would draw the line. Now we will see whether our guidance all through the years pays off or not. Even if your children decide to get to this level of intimacy during adolescence, thanks to all your preparation they will act wisely and responsibly and their risk of harm will be minimized. But don't judge your success as an approachable parent solely on whether your children engage in intimate sexual behavior or not—judge it more on your child's ability to act responsibly in the face of temptation and inherent risk. Even if you would prefer that your child does not go this far as a teen, if he does he will have a better chance of keeping himself safe if you have done your job as an approachable parent.

If your child does become involved in some intimate touching under the clothes, you may be all right with that if it's done with someone your child deeply trusts and respects—ideally, someone with good character and judgment, someone you and your partner or spouse have met and approve of. We parents can at least hope our child has already formed a fairly solid bond with the chosen partner.

Sexual Intercourse and Other Types of Intercourse

Based on the best available statistics, just about half of all teens in this country have had sexual intercourse.[1] So, statistically, there's a good chance that your child will engage in intercourse at least once while still a teenager. However, if you follow the guidelines laid out in this book, this will likely *not* be the case. I'm assuming it's your goal to ensure that your child will not have sex as a teen and that he will avoid the primary sexual risk behaviors that represent some of the major causes of illness and death in this country. When I advocate delaying intercourse until adulthood I make the assumption that, all things being equal, a person is more likely to behave responsibly as an adult than as a teen. I fully understand that there are many adults who behave irresponsibly and make their fair share of mistakes. It is just that with teenagers, from a developmental standpoint, they are still learning the basic concept that present behavior has future consequences. That is, many still lack the ability to see beyond their noses.

However, if your teenager does become sexually active, our goal is that it be with someone with whom she has mutual love, respect, and trust. You know I have some reservations about just how good our kids are at identifying real love, even with all of our approachable guidance. Yet I hope the big three will be a part of their decision to go ahead and have sex, if they make that choice.

Thanks to all of the work you are putting into being an approachable parent, your child will still be making far better decisions than if you had remained on the sidelines all these years. Don't forget this. *Without* your efforts to be approachable, think what your child *might* have gotten involved in with respect to sex.

Dating and Getting Involved

At what age do you think it's okay for your child to start to date and get seriously involved with a boyfriend or girlfriend? Are you okay with your kid forming some sort of romantic relationship during high school? How about during middle school? You will need to come to terms with your expectations for your children.

When I visit fifth-grade classrooms, I am struck by the number of kids who appear to be engaging in some form of dating. It may not be the classically defined "couple date" but it does involve some pairing off in various social situations. Irrespective of how one defines dating, going out, hanging out, hooking up, or getting involved, our kids will likely form "romantic" relationships in one form or another.

I recommend that you address this issue with your child proactively, around age ten, before she or he gets to middle school. By starting your conversations around ten years of age, you start to lay the groundwork for establishing boundaries that you hope your child will abide down the road. This means sharing your thoughts and expectations about dating or get-togethers that are different from regular socials with one's friends and peers. I don't think kids in middle school need to be dating or even thinking about forming a special relationship with another. I think they are too young and it restricts their ability to branch out and explore the social landscape. Having said that, I do think that it's important that your child take advantage of as many socializing opportunities as possible in order to make friends and gain experience interacting with others.

Hazards Online

It is here where you also want to hammer home the potential pitfalls of the Internet. Numerous hazards await your child online, whether he is surfing the Internet or joins the online social networking scene. I know I spoke about these hazards earlier but I want to take another moment to have you reflect on how important it is that you discourage your child's involvement. You know the reality behind social networking and unsupervised online Internet surfing. Nothing, I repeat, nothing is more important on the social landscape issue than having your child meet and interact with others *in person*. Sitting in front of a computer screen does not take the place of real face-to-face involvement with other people (not to mention the importance of being active physically). And I'll throw the whole texting thing in there as well. You know our children spend way too much time on these high-tech activities and not enough time actually interacting socially with their peers. And when you throw in the potential destructiveness of harassment, bullying, and exposure to uncensored material that can come with being online and involved with social networks, this activity becomes even more dangerous. You must find the strength to limit your child's participation. Specifically, supervise your kid when he's on the Internet until at least high school, and forbid him from joining the social network scene until, well, adulthood.

Many parents will disagree with me, especially with respect to social networking. Your kids may be participating right now on a social networking site. Some of them might still be in elementary school. For all the supposed benefits of the social network scene, people reaching out and connecting to a diverse, eclectic, and expanded social environment, we know all too well that it has a downside that can be devastating and deadly. At the very least, it is not a place for eleven-, twelve-, or thirteen-year-old children to be; plain and simple.

It's in the Script

As your child begins to expand her awareness of in-person social opportunities in middle school, you can introduce to her the idea of scripting her outings. That is, prior to your child going out with peers, you and she develop a script of what is expected to occur on the outing—much as a movie script determines how the characters interact and what actually occurs in a scene. This includes when the outing starts and the time it will conclude, who will be at the outing, what happens if someone suggests a change in the plans, and the time you want your child to check in with you. Doing this with your child establishes clear expectations and boundaries for her social get-togethers and will be a useful tool to use when she actually starts to date. It forces her to think about being responsible while out with others, especially when you have her reflect on her course of action in the event that someone tries to change what was planned for the outing. This happens all the time, doesn't it? The kids have plans, they go out, and suddenly someone wants to do something different. Changes of plans can get our kids in trouble so make sure your child always lets you know when it comes up.

You can see how much easier it would be to discuss your reservations about middle school dating prior to the actual middle school years. If there is one central theme that I've harped on this entire book, it is the need to have conversations about important issues *before* your child starts to experience them. And dating is no different. You sure don't want to start your conversations about it when your seventh- or eighth-grade child comes home from school one day and tells you he'd like to go out on a date tonight. Trust me; you don't want to have to scramble and improvise.

Keeping the Conversations Going

Middle school will be an altogether different experience from elementary school for both you and your child. Somewhere during this time your kid is going to start to pull back from you. Fortunately for you, your attempts at being approachable all these years will pay off handsomely. I speak to a lot of middle school parent groups and I always cringe inside when a parent tells me that he really hasn't dealt with sex and sexuality to date and now wants to know how to proceed. I always say better late than never but in all likelihood he has a pretty steep hill to climb as he moves forward in his efforts to become approachable. You, on the other hand, as a result of reading this book, will be way ahead of the game by the time

What Your Child Needs to Know About Sex (and When)

your children get to the sixth grade. Yet, even though you may have done a good job up to now, you must keep things going. You have to stay on top of your game at all times when it comes to being approachable.

You'll need to remember that sexual feelings will continue to become a more pervasive reality for your child, becoming more recognizable in middle school and far more relevant in high school. Consequently, you will want to continue your conversations, authentic teachings, and setting of boundaries on how to manage and deal with this part of your child's sexuality. Continue to be supportive of your child's sexual feelings, yet remind him of the risks of being sexually active and the need to have love, respect, and trust as part of a relationship. Your child is a sexual human being, and by acknowledging his sexual feelings you will help him to feel normal. Your child's middle school and even high school years will bring alternating episodes of both maturity and childish behavior that at times will keep you guessing about who your kid really is. But that is the way it is with a middle-school and early-high-school child—your kids are still kids even though they're becoming more and more like adults.

By middle school, puberty will be in full bloom and your child will be going through so many changes physically and emotionally that you need to be as laid back with it all as is possible. Keep making occasional references that the changes he's going through are normal and feel free to jump in at any point to help him better understand those changes. Unlike when you started your puberty discussions way back when your child was in elementary school, your child is now living and breathing puberty every day. Be prepared, though; some children don't change as quickly as their peers, and if your child's in sixth grade or early seventh grade, he may not be changing much at all. You will need to reassure him that changes are indeed on their way if he just sits tight and stays the course.

I let my own son know that my puberty changes didn't start until midway through seventh grade. This was back in the day when every student had to shower after gym class, and on the very first day of class I noticed that there was a big difference between my body and the other boys' bodies when I stripped down to shower. "Wow," I thought to myself, "there are some pretty big penises in here and many of them have a lot of hair around them." I, on the other hand, didn't have a single pubic hair and as far as my penis went, well, let's just say it was still a little fellow. I made up my mind that very first day of school to avoid the showers as best I could, or I would hide out in the locker room until the other guys finished and then dart in for a quick wash. Needless to say, I was late for my next class on numerous occasions. But as it turned out, all of my worrying was for naught; as it wasn't too long after these experiences that I started to go through puberty. At long last, I started to fit in a whole lot better. A story or two like this can be very helpful if you've got a child who's lagging behind.

Overall, you will be balancing your involvement as an approachable sex educator for the next seven or so years by speaking up when it's really important and laying back when things aren't quite as pressing. You can't talk your teenager to death but you can't avoid her either. Using teachable moments will be very helpful, as they can be used as a springboard into a brief conversation that won't feel as contrived as a formal sit-down discussion would. Be smart about choosing those times when you do have a one-on-one with your child. Riding in the car, bike riding, or taking a subway with your kid can give you some moments to chat without interruption and won't be viewed by your child as one of those formal talk moments.

Try not to get frustrated if your teen doesn't respond much when you talk to him or her. Many parents of middle and high school age kids complain about this during my presentations with them. "My kid just doesn't want to talk to me anymore, Dr. Fred," they worry. "No matter what I do I just can't get them to say much to me." It's okay. Our teenagers are not supposed to talk too much to us. That is just the way it is when you get to this age. They are no longer those cute little talkative kids they were just a few years earlier.

So you'll have to get over it and move on; there's no use wishing for something that at least for now just doesn't exist anymore. When your kid reaches his junior or senior year in high school he will begin to morph back into the wonderful kid you remember him to be. Maturity will do that to most kids. But for now what does count most is that you continue to be approachable and find those times to speak up and say to your child what you think needs to be said. If your kids complain and bitch about your involvement, you can reply, "Too bad; it's because I love you so much that I have to say what I say." Your kids may not show it, but they love it when you tell them you love them; it gets them every time!

Alcohol, Drugs, and Sex

The reality of alcohol, drugs, and sex for teens today in our country is alarming. More than 20 percent of kids in this country have had a significant drinking episode before age thirteen. That's one in five kids! In addition, more than 20 percent of kids who are sexually active used alcohol or drugs the last time they had sexual intercourse.[2] You'll recall that sexual risk behaviors are one of six health-related behaviors that account for the majority of major illness and death in our country. Well, alcohol and substance use is another one of those six major health behaviors. Each of these behaviors is dangerous enough by itself. But together, sexual risk behaviors *and* alcohol and drug use are positively deadly. We must wake up about the potentially lethal combination of the two among young people. Getting high and having sex can be a deadly combination. In addition, getting high can open the door to other potentially harmful behaviors. Statistically, significant risk behaviors such as using alcohol and illegal drugs and substances are behind the majority of serious crimes in this country and a major cause of vehicle-related accidents and deaths.

When teens get high they risk compromising their ability to make reasonable and responsible decisions. Put them in a social situation when they are intoxicated, and of course the risk of engaging in sexual behavior becomes more real. It is not just the risk of engaging in intercourse but also the risk of not using a condom or becoming sexually active with multiple partners. We must be aware of the significant problems associated with teen drinking and drugging and sexual activity, and help our kids understand how to minimize their risk for engaging in all of these behaviors, both by themselves and when done together.

I hope you have already had conversations with your child about the hazards of drinking and misusing drugs, both legal and illegal ones. At around the time your child is about to enter middle school, age eleven or so, have your first talks about the risks and dangers of mixing alcohol and drug use with sexual activity. Talk about how, even if you're not interested in sex, alcohol and drugs can break down your inhibitions. These hazards are real. It's very likely that your children and mine will try alcohol and some legal or illegal substances prior to graduating from high school. We deceive ourselves when we think, *Oh, not my child.* Remember, most of us tend to underestimate what our children are involved with.

I think your conversations about drinking and using drugs should happen periodically throughout middle school. Several times each year, check in with your kid and remind him of your expectations around making good decisions as they apply to these issues. You can use the same strategies for dealing with alcohol and drugs that you have used for sex and sexuality; teachable moments, authentic teaching, and using the media are all useful when dealing with the topics of alcohol, drugs, and sex, or with any other critical health issue, for that matter.

I am constantly asked by parents how often or how many times should they bring a particular subject up with their kids. I hate to put a number on these things, but I would say that you should devote at least one major conversation each year during the middle school years that link together alcohol, drugs, and sex, and perhaps more often depending on each of your own particular situations. A reminder or two before your child goes out somewhere with her friends won't hurt. Don't beat a dead horse, but do justice to this important issue. When it comes to your child's health and safety, there are many such issues. Certainly, as your child gets older, enters high school, and expands her opportunities to encounter more and varied social situations, you will probably increase the number of discussions you have with her around these topics.

Too Permissive or Too Strict?

As I've discussed earlier, an *authoritative* style of parenting, from an empirical standpoint, is the most effective style—not too strict and not too permissive. Operate by a clearly established set of rules and boundaries, identify a set of rights and wrongs, and allow room for input and discussion—these are the basics of effective parenting.

But what if you're too permissive with your child? Or just the opposite: way too strict? I have come across more than my share of both types, and each presents its own unique set of difficulties for parents who are trying to handle a hormonally charged teenager.

Let's Be Friends

As I've said before, permissive parents want to be friends with their kids. They allow their teens to drink in the home and allow their kid's girlfriend or boyfriend to have more than their share of privacy and alone time in the house. You'll see them allow the girlfriend or boyfriend to stay overnight occasionally, and even allow them to sleep in their child's room. They don't want any confrontation with their children; they give them way too much leeway. They will supply their teenager with condoms but not spend a whole lot of time in meaningful discussion about core values and sexuality (see sidebar).

The inherent flaw in a permissive parent's thinking is that a minor child has the personal right to make her own decisions about sex, so the parent's wishes take a backseat to the child's. Although the permissive parent may not want her teenager to date until a certain age, or become too serious with a girlfriend or boyfriend until after high school, or fool around early in adolescence, this parent will abandon any of these wishes and cave to her child's demands.

My Way or the Highway

At the other extreme, the authoritarian style parent is really not any better at things either. The authoritarian parent doesn't want his kid doing any fooling around. There isn't a whole lot of room for discussion; if what the kid wants goes against what the parent wants, then forget it. There's no middle ground. This dictatorial style doesn't hold together well at all during adolescence. Fear of punishment may at first discourage a child from acting a certain way, but over the long haul the child is going to rebel. Punishment will have no long-lasting, positive influence on the child. The older the child grows, the more difficult it becomes to control him. The fear of punishment that the child felt when he was younger is replaced with anger as he grows older, and that anger drives him to act contrary to what his parent wants. So if it's abstinence that the parent wants, it'll be sexual intercourse that the parent gets. What better way to get back at a hurtful parent than to do the very thing the parent doesn't want you to do?

We see kids rebelling under this sort of parental regime by sexually acting out when they get the chance. The teenager of this sort of parent eventually does all he can do to get away with things when his parent isn't looking or paying attention.

THE PERMISSIVE PARENT

A permissive parent came up to me after one of my presentations and we had the following brief conversation.

"I gave my thirteen-year-old daughter a condom," she told me, confident that I would be impressed.

"Oh, really," I replied, "and what sort of discussion did you have with her?"

The parent said, "'In case you ever have sex I want to just make sure that you are prepared.'"

"And what else did you say to her?"

"Well, um, you see, I really didn't want to get into too much talk because I didn't want to say anything that maybe she wouldn't like to hear."

This is the perfect example of the permissive parent. A noble intention, wanting her daughter to be able to protect herself should she have sexual intercourse, but the parent provided no parental oversight. She could have shared with her daughter her thoughts about sexual intercourse, and when and with whom it should be engaged in, and the exchange would have been much more effective.

You just don't hand over a condom to a thirteen-year-old without having a major conversation beforehand. The parent acted as if her daughter was just a friend of hers who was about to have sex but forgot to bring protection. ("Oh, here you go, take one of my condoms, I've got plenty more.") But when the person is her thirteen-year-old daughter and the parent behaves this way, what message is she sending? Rather than setting boundaries that discourage sexual intercourse and having meaningful two-way discussions about why these boundaries are in a thirteen-year-old girl's best interests, this parent acted as if she didn't want to infringe on her daughter's personal right of sexual expression.

A Sexually Responsible Adolescent

We've dealt with so many aspects of sex and sexuality, haven't we? We explored in detail how to become an approachable parent on all matters that are sexual, beginning early in life and continuing right through childhood. Our goal: to provide the necessary knowledge and guidance that will assist our children to develop into healthy and responsible sexual adolescents. And here we are! On the cusp of having our teenager go out and successfully negotiate a sexualized world, and emerging ready and able to take on the challenges of adulthood. You have the power to make it all work for your kids. If you carefully follow what I've laid out here for you, your child will weather adolescence in a way that we hope for. You will have prepared your child to handle his emerging sexuality in a way that he will understand and accept, and by being approachable you will remain at his side, serving as both parent and mentor.

Your Goals, Revisited

Let's take some time now and go over what we expect to have accomplished by the time our child is well on her way through adolescence. The following list represents what I would consider the fruits of your labor in becoming an approachable parent for any sexual issue or situation. Your adolescent will:

- *Be comfortable with his or her sexual identity.* You will want your adolescent to be comfortable in his or her own skin, being male or female. However your children come to define their femaleness or their maleness, they will be at ease with who and what they are. This means being at ease with their sexual orientation, comfortable in knowing what that orientation entails, and secure in knowing that their parents accept and acknowledge who and what they are.

- *Have a healthy body image.* Your adolescent will accept what she or he looks like and will be responsible in maintaining and caring for her or his physical self.
- *Have a good understanding of puberty and the physical changes that occur with it.* Your adolescent will be comfortable when you discuss information about puberty and will come to you when your guidance is needed.
- *Appreciate that physical changes are normal.*
- *Have a good awareness of the characteristics that make for a caring, loving person.* Your adolescent will see the value of these characteristics in forming friendships and relationships.
- *Demonstrate an awareness of what love, respect, and trust is and how they manifest themselves in a romantic relationship with another.* We've discussed so much the importance of these qualities in a relationship that you will want to continue to extol their virtues throughout your child's adolescence.
- *Understand that sexual feelings are normal and can be very powerful.*
- *Appreciate the importance of having love, respect, and trust in a relationship before having sexual intercourse.*
- *Avoid sexual intercourse until fully mature.*
- *Avoid unplanned pregnancy.*
- *Avoid abusive romantic relationships.*
- *Avoid sexually transmitted infections.*

You've worked hard to convince your child of the importance of delaying sexual intercourse and intimate sexual touching until she or he has love, respect, and trust in a relationship—and ideally not until she or he is an adult. But again, if your adolescent does have intercourse while in high school, you should not consider this a failure. Your adolescent is allowed to make mistakes; it is after all one of the things that makes us distinctly human. Through it all, I think you want to judge whether or not you are a successful, approachable parent based on your adolescent's ability to make responsible sexual decisions, and, if he is in a relationship, how he treats the other person. It is so important for an adolescent to know how to treat others. Not having to worry that my child might be nasty to others or choose a partner who would be unkind toward him is very important to me, and I'm sure you feel the same way. Of course, making good, responsible decisions is too.

Conclusion

If there is just one thing you can take away from reading this book, I would like it to be the fact that you can be the single most influential source of sexual information and guidance in your children's lives. If you can establish yourself as an approachable parent on all matters related to sex, you will minimize the chances that your child will engage in sexually related behavior that is dangerous to her or his health and safety. No other source of sex education is more powerful or more effective than you—none! If you take the initiative to make an early start in your conversations about sex and sexuality, and follow the steps outlined here, your children will be in the best position possible to develop into sexually healthy and responsible adolescents and young adults.

Don't be afraid to become and remain actively involved in the sex education of your children. You must stay in charge. Remember that your kids are being educated and potentially influenced every day by a sex-saturated society that is relentless in its pursuit to confuse and distort your children's understanding of what it means to be male and female. If you sit back and allow it, this sexualized world will swallow your children whole, and by the time they reach adolescence they will be primed to behave sexually in ways that are contrary to their best interests. The Internet, the social networking world, your children's peers, and the vastly sexualized media never take a day off. Day in and day out, all of these forces influence your children, and without your intervention and guidance they will have harmful effects on their lives.

This is a battle, and it is one that you could lose. In research, most kids say that they don't receive enough guidance from their parents on sexual matters.[3] This should not be a surprise since a majority of parents are either uncomfortable talking about sex, would rather have someone else teach their children about sex, or are afraid that talking about it will cause their kids to become too interested in it. So if you are one of these parents, then your children will be influenced about sex more from outside sources than from you. And if that is to happen, your children will pay the price.

But all you need to do is to become approachable, and you will win the battle. Think positively and optimistically as you move forward. What an awesome set of responsibilities you have, caring for the most precious thing in your life: your children. Parenting is certainly the most difficult and complex thing you will ever do; to also be the primary sexual educator for your children makes it that much more difficult. Your parents and your grandparents didn't have to be the sexual educators that you have to be today, and there was no one to teach you how to prepare for all the sexually charged topics that you now have to help your kids understand. But the way things are in our society nowadays demands that you actively educate your children about sex and sexuality on a regular and ongoing basis. There isn't much room to slack off.

Your children need you to be the go-to person on all things sexual. There is no escaping that reality. Now is the time to step up and be that person. You can do it. Let's all join together and make sure that we, our children's parents, become the most important and significant source of sexual guidance in our children's lives. When we do this, our children will be the winners.

Good luck!

NOTES

Chapter 1

1. P. Bearman and H. Brückner, "Peer Effects on Adolescent Sexual Debut and Pregnancy: An Analysis of a National Survey of Adolescent Girls," The National Campaign to Prevent Teen Pregnancy, in *Peer Potential: Making the Most of How Teens Influence Each Other* (Washington, DC: National Campaign to Prevent Teen Pregnancy, April 1999): 7–26; J. D. Brown, K. L. L'Engle, C. J. Pardun, G. Guo, K. Kenneavy, and C. Jackson, "Sexy Media Matter: Exposure to Sexual Content in Music, Movies, Television, and Magazines Predicts Black and White Adolescents' Sexual Behavior," *Pediatrics* 117 (April 2006): 1018–1027; V. C. Strasburger and the Council on Communications and Media, "Sexuality, Contraception, and the Media," *Pediatrics* 126 (September 2010): 576–582.

2. B. Albert, *With One Voice 2010: America's Adults and Teens Sound Off about Teen Pregnancy* (Washington, DC: The National Campaign to Prevent Teen and Unplanned Pregnancy, 2010).

3. M. E. Eisenberg, D. H. Bernat, L. H. Bearinger, and M. D. Resnick, "Support for Comprehensive Sexuality Education: Perspectives from Parents of School-Age Youth," *Journal of Adolescent Health* 42, no. 4 (April 2008): 352–359; Hickman-Brown Public Opinion Research, "Public Support for Sexuality Education Reaches Highest Levels" (Washington, DC: Advocates for Youth, 1999); D. J. Landry, S. Singh and J. E. Darroch,

"Sexuality Education in Fifth and Sixth Grades in U.S. Public Schools, 1999," *Family Planning Perspectives* 32, no. 5 (September/October 2000): 212–219; National Public Radio, Kaiser Family Foundation, and Kennedy School of Government, "Sex Education in America: General Public/ Parents Survey" (January 2004), http://www.kff.org/newsmedia/upload/ Sex-Education-in-America-Summary.pdf.

4. American Association of University Women, *Hostile Hallways: The AAUW Survey on Sexual Harassment in America's Schools* (Washington, DC: AAUW Educational Foundation, 1993).

Chapter 2

1. S. Elliott, "Parents' Constructions of Teen Sexuality: Sex Panics, Contradictory Discourses, and Social Inequality," *Symbolic Interaction* 33, no. 2 (2010): 191–212; L. O'Donnell, A. Stueve, R. Duran, A. Myint-U, G. Agronick, A. San Doval, and R. Wilson-Simmons, "Parenting Practices, Parents' Underestimation of Daughters' Risks, and Alcohol and Sexual Behaviors of Urban Girls," *Journal of Adolescent Health* 42, no. 5 (May 2008): 496–502.

2. D. Baumrind, "Child Care Practices Anteceding Three Patterns of Preschool Behavior," *Genetic Psychology Monographs* 75, no.1 (1967): 43–88; E. E. Maccoby and J. A. Martin, "Socialization in the Context of the Family: Parent–Child Interaction," in P. H. Mussen and E. M. Hetherington, *Handbook of Child Psychology: Socialization, Personality, and Social Development (Volume 4)* (New York: Wiley, 1983): 1–102.

3. Centers for Disease Control and Prevention, "Youth Risk Behavior Surveillance—United States, 2009," *Surveillance Summaries* 59, no. SS-5 (MMWR: 2010).

4. C. M. Markham, S. R. Tortolero, S. L. Escobar-Chaves, G. S. Parcel, R. Harrist, and R. C. Addy, "Family Connectedness and Sexual Risk-Taking Among Urban Youth Attending Alternative High Schools," *Perspectives on Sexual and Reproductive Health* 35, no. 4 (July/August 2003): 174–179; M. D. Resnick and P. M. Rinehart, *Influencing Behavior: The Power of Protective Factors in Reducing Youth Violence* (Minneapolis: Division of General Pediatrics and Adolescent Health, University of Minnesota Adolescent Health Program, 2004).

Chapter 3

1. M. D. Stein, K. A. Freedberg, L. M. Sullivan, J. Savetsky, S. M. Levenson, R. Hingson, and J. H. Samet, "Sexual Ethics: Disclosure of HIV-Positive Status to Partners," *Archives of Internal Medicine* 158, no. 3 (February 1998): 253–257.

Chapter 4

1. G. Ryan, T. Leversee, and S. Lane, eds., *Juvenile Sexual Offending* (San Francisco: Jossey-Bass, 2007).

2. F. Kaeser, C. DiSalvo, and R. Moglia, "Sexual Behaviors of Young Children that Occur in Schools," *Journal of Sex Education and Therapy* 25, no. 4 (2000): 277–285.

3. Centers for Disease Control and Prevention, "Youth Risk Behavior Surveillance—United States, 2009," *Surveillance Summaries* 59, no. SS-5 (MMWR: 2010).

4. A. Chandra, W. D. Mosher, C. Copen, and C. Sionean, "Sexual Behavior, Sexual Attraction, and Sexual Identity in the United States: Data from the 2006–2008 National Survey of Family Growth," *National Center for Health Statistics* 36 (March 2011).

Chapter 6

1. Centers for Disease Control and Prevention, "Youth Risk Behavior Surveillance—United States, 2009," *Surveillance Summaries* 59, no. SS-5 (MMWR: 2010).

2. Ibid.

Chapter 7

1. N. M. Malamuth, T. Addison, and J. Koss, "Pornography and Sexual Aggression: Are there Reliable Effects and Can We Understand Them?" *Annual Review of Sex Research* 11 (2000): 26–94; V. Vega and N. M. Malamuth, "Predicting Sexual Aggression: The Role of Pornography in the Context of General and Specific Risk Factors," *Aggressive Behavior* 33, no. 2 (March/April 2007): 104–117.

Chapter 8

1. F. M. Biro, M. P. Galvez, L. C. Greenspan, P. A. Succop, N. Van-geepuram, S. M. Pinney, S. Teitelbaum, G. C. Windham, L. H. Kushi, and M. S. Wolff, "Pubertal Assessment Method and Baseline Characteristics in a Mixed Longitudinal Study of Girls," *Pediatrics* 126, no. 3 (September 2010): 583–90; F. O. Finlay, R. Jones, and J. Coleman, "Is Puberty Getting Earlier? The Views of Doctors and Teachers," *Child: Care, Health and Development* 28, no. 3 (May 2002): 205–9.

2. Centers for Disease Control and Prevention, "Youth Risk Behavior Surveillance—United States, 2009," *Surveillance Summaries* 59, no. SS-5 (MMWR: 2010).

3. Centers for Disease Control and Prevention, "Youth Risk Behavior Surveillance—United States, 2009," *Surveillance Summaries* 59, no. SS-5 (MMWR: 2010); J. G. Silverman, A. Raj, L. A. Mucci, and J. E.

Hathaway, "Dating Violence Against Adolescent Girls and Associated Substance Use, Unhealthy Weight Control, Sexual Risk Behavior, Pregnancy, and Suicidality," *Journal of the American Medical Association* 286, no. 5 (2001): 572–579.

4. Centers for Disease Control and Prevention, "Youth Risk Behavior Surveillance—United States, 2009," *Surveillance Summaries* 59, no. SS-5 (MMWR: 2010).

5. Guttmacher Institute, "Facts on Induced Abortion in the United States, In Brief" (New York: Guttmacher, 2011), http://www.guttmacher.org/pubs/fb induced abortion.html. Accessed February 15, 2011.

Chapter 9

1. Centers for Disease Control and Prevention, "Youth Risk Behavior Surveillance—United States, 2009," *Surveillance Summaries* 59, no. SS-5 (MMWR: 2010).

2. Ibid.

3. B. Albert, *With One Voice 2010: America's Adults and Teens Sound Off about Teen Pregnancy* (Washington, DC: The National Campaign to Prevent Teen and Unplanned Pregnancy, 2010).

ABOUT THE AUTHOR

DR. FRED KAESER has been a sexual educator and director of health for more than twenty-five years in the largest public school system in America, the New York City public schools. He developed the first student sexual harassment policy for the NYC Department of Education and has spoken on sexuality throughout the United States and Canada. Currently, Dr. Kaeser remains a consultant for the NYC Department of Education. He has a doctoral degree in human sexuality from New York University, where he still teaches. He lives with his family in Centerport, NY.

INDEX

on sexual feelings, 143, 175–76
sharing values about life and
sexuality, 33–37
telling a story, 55–56
Authoritarian parenting style, 28, 196
Authoritative parenting style, 5, 28, 38

B

Bad aspects of sex
helping children avoid, 73–74
online harassment, 65
overview, 59–60
sexual bullying, 64–70, 71
targeting specific sexualities, 65–70
teenage pregnancy, 47, 74
teenage sexual intercourse, 71–72,
186–87
Bath time, monitoring, 27
Birth control. *See* Abstinence; Condoms
Bisexuals, 65–66
Body image, 134, 149, 152, 199
Body parts. *See* Private parts
Bonding with your child, 37–38
Books on sex, using, 93
Boundaries, setting, 5, 34–37, 190, 195
Breasts
answering child's questions about,
86–87
development during puberty, 129, 135
making fun of, 179–80
privacy of, 81–82

C

Circumcision, 135
Clitoris, 81, 118, 120, 124
Community-based organizations, 18
Computers, monitoring access to, 26
Condoms
for HIV protection, 37, 163, 166
how to use, 140, 165–67

Contraception, 139
Curiosity, sexual, 22, 68

D

Dating and getting involved
adolescents, 187–88
decision-making scenarios, 179
discussing before middle school
years, 190
Decision-making, 92–93, 178–81
Dildos, 14, 25, 164
Dressing sexy, 37, 75, 108
Drugs and alcohol, 141, 193–95

E

Egg cells, 80, 88
Eight-year-olds
discouraging the use of slang, 91–92
discussing masturbation, 120
discussing puberty with, 138, 146,
147–51
discussing sexual intercourse, 45, 99,
146, 154–58
learning about HIV, 74, 158
learning sexual modesty, 81
sexual topics to discuss with, 88–89
starting puberty, 129
talking about sex with, 98–99
Ejaculation, 121, 136, 137
Elementary school children. *See also*
specific age groups
on the cusp of puberty, 5
sex education lacking for, 16–17
sexualized behavior in, 14–15
Eleven-year-olds, 5, 72, 100
Empathy, learning, 42, 107, 108
Erections, 135, 150, 151

F

Fantasy, during masturbation, 127, 128
Feeling up and down over the clothes, 185
Feeling up and down under the clothes, 186
Fifth graders. *See also* Ten-year-olds
  dating, 188
  developmental changes in, 151–52
  discussing homosexuality with, 110
  leaving fifth grade and entering
    middle school, 144
Five-year-olds
  sexual bullying and, 65
  sexual curiosity of, 22
  sexualized behavior in, 22–23
  talking about sex with, 101–4
  touching private parts, 73
Five-year-olds, learning about
  function of body parts, 87–88
  HIV, 33
  homosexuality, 33–34
  love, respect, and trust, 44–45
  making a baby, 44–45
  private parts, 82–83, 87–88
  sexual intercourse, 99, 101–2
Foreskin, 135
Four-year-olds
  answering questions about private
    parts, 85–88
  knowing the names for private
    parts, 81
  touching private parts, 73
Friends. *See also* Peer group
  best friends versus ordinary friends,
    50–51
  developing over time, 52–53
  knowing your child's friends, 26,
    144–45
  learning love, respect, and trust
    through, 56
  reasons for breaking off, 49
  teaching your child about, 108

G

Gays and lesbians
  being comfortable with one's sexual
    identity, 198–99
  children as, 167–69
  discrimination against, 65–66
  marriage and, 105
  parenting issues, 101, 102, 122
  teaching children about, 109–11, 164
Genitals. *See also* Private parts
  ignorance about, 79–80
  slang words for, 78–81
  touching, 14, 84
  touching others, 64, 69
Goals of approachable parenting, 198–99
Good aspects of sex, 60–62. *See also*
    Love, respect, and trust

H

Hair growth, during puberty, 134
Hairstyles, 108
High school students. *See also*
    Adolescents; Teenagers
  alcohol and drug use, 141
  feeling up and down over the
    clothes, 185
  having sexual intercourse, 140,
    199–200
HIV
  condoms protecting from, 37, 140,
    163, 166
  discussing with five-year-olds, 33
  discussing with nine- or ten-year-old,
    46, 163
  eight-year-olds learning about, 74, 158
  partner not disclosing, 46
  transmitting through sexual
    intercourse, 75, 140, 158, 163

Homosexuality. *See also* Gays and
lesbians
being comfortable with one's sexual
identity, 198–99
discussing with your child, 33–34,
109–11
Hormones, during puberty, 134, 138
Hygiene, personal, 153
Hypersexualization, 1–2, 9, 13–15

I

"I'll show you mine if you show me
yours" game, 68
Infatuation, love versus, 48
Insemination, artificial, 105
Internet. *See also* Social networking sites
hazards of using, 188–89
screening and monitoring, 27, 127–28
sexual intercourse viewed on, 7–8

J

Journaling, 55

K

Kindergarten children, 98–100. *See also*
Five-year-olds
Kissing, 184–85

L

Letter writing, 175
Life partner, choosing, 106–7
Love, respect, and trust. *See also* Values
adolescent's awareness of, 199
authentic instruction on, 55–57, 143
importance of, 41–42
misunderstanding true love, 47
modeling, 57
overview, 57–58

power of, 42–44
real-life examples of, 45–46, 52, 54
recognizing, 48–49, 51–54, 61–62
talking with your child about, 44–47
teenager's sexual partner and, 187
in true friendships, 49–51
Lovemaking aspect of sexual
intercourse, 79
Lust, love versus, 48
Lyrics, demeaning, 8, 90, 172–73

M

Making a baby, 44–45, 88, 157–58.
See also Sexual intercourse
Marriage, 105
Masturbation. *See also* Orgasm
benefits of, 113–14, 115–16
boys versus girls, 133
described, 136–37
excessive, 122–24
guilt over, 114, 117
infants and, 117, 133
instructing your child about, 120–21
learning through practice, 117–19
mutual, 125
parents disapproving, 114–16
parents sending affirmative
messages about, 117
with peers, 118–19
pornography and fantasy with, 126–28
teachable moments, 117
time and place for, 116
Menstruation
beginning of, 129
describing, 136
discussing with your daughter,
133, 148–49
importance of understanding, 92
mean ages for, 100

Middle school children.
    See also Adolescents
    dating and getting involved, 188
    discussing alcohol and drugs, 194–95
    entering middle school, 144
    feeling up and down over the clothes,
        185
    keeping conversations going, 190–93
    kissing, 184
    sexual behavior of, 183
Modeling, 57
Modesty, sexual, 81, 122
Music lyrics, demeaning, 8, 90, 172–73

N

Nine-year-olds, learning about
    abortion, 161
    condoms, 164–67
    gays and lesbians, 164
    HIV, 46, 163
    masturbation, 120
    oral and anal sex, 162–64
    puberty, 137–38, 151–54
    sexual behavior, 159
    sexual feelings, 173–76
    sexual intercourse, 46, 154–61
Ninth graders, pregnancy rate in, 74
Nipples, changes during puberty, 135
Normal, helping child feel, 132, 152
Nudity, 81, 84–85

O

Oral sex
    discussing with nine- and ten-year-
        olds, 162–64
    explaining to six-year-olds, 96–97
    misconceptions about, 162
    prevalence of, 75
    as sex, 74–75, 139
    values statement about, 37

Orgasm
    describing, 124–25
    infants having, 133
    pornography's help with, 126
    ten-year-olds knowledge of, 122–23,
        124
Ovaries, 80, 88
Ovulation, 92, 135–36, 139, 148–49

P

Parenting
    authoritarian, 28, 196
    authoritative, 5, 28, 38
    effective, 27–28, 195
    lack of education on, 63
    permissive, 28, 29, 195–96, 197
    uninvolved, 28
Parents
    becoming comfortable talking with
        your child, 141–42
    communicating with teenagers,
        192–93
    counteracting damaging sexual
        messages, 20–23
    doubts about talking to child about
        sex, 4–5
    gay and lesbian, 101, 102, 122
    goals for adolescents, 198–200
    monitoring child's life and world,
        26–28
    as primary sex educator for their
        child, 2, 18, 93, 191–92, 200–201
    remaining silent versus taking a
        stand, 11–13
    sexual messages from, 11
    single, 122
Passion, love versus, 48
Pedophiles, 127